Rob Temple is a journalist and founder of the Very British Problems (@SoVeryBritish) social media feeds, which now have more than five million followers, and a consultant on the official Channel 4 Very British Problems series.

Originally from Peterborough, he now lives in Cambridge with his collection of jackets and his thoughts.

D1325275

ROB TEMPLE

BORN TO BE MILD

ADVENTURES FOR THE ANXIOUS

sphere

SPHERE

First published in Great Britain in 2020 by Sphere
This paperback edition published by Sphere in 2021

1 3 5 7 9 10 8 6 4 2

A CIP catalogue record for this book
is available from the British Library.

ISBN 978-0-7515-7473-9

Typeset in Caslon by M Rules
Printed and bound in Great Britain by
Clays Ltd, Elcograf S.p.A.

Papers used by Sphere are from well-managed forests
and other responsible sources.

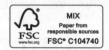

MIX
Paper from
responsible sources
FSC® C104740

Sphere
An imprint of
Little, Brown Book Group
Carmelite House
50 Victoria Embankment
London EC4Y 0DZ

An Hachette UK Company
www.hachette.co.uk

www.littlebrown.co.uk

For Mum and Dad

Went to see Rob Roy's grave.
Saw it, came back.

The Secret Diary of Adrian Mole, Aged 13¾
SUE TOWNSEND

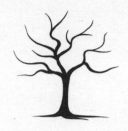

A FOREWORD BY BARACK OBAMA

... would be good, wouldn't it? Couldn't get him, unfortunately.

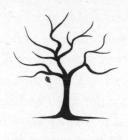

INTRODUCTION

'Ooh, baby, baby, it's a mild world'.
'Mild thing, you make my heart sing'.
'Hey, babe, take a walk on the mild side'.
'Mild horses couldn't drag me away'.
'BORN... TO BE... MII–III–LD!'

What do these lyrics have in common? That's right, they don't exist. The wild and reckless get to be in rock songs, not us: the mild and feckless. But can mild people (those timid worrywarts who carry reserve umbrellas in case the main umbrella fails to deploy) still be adventurers? Is it possible to get the same kicks traditionally enjoyed whizzing down Route 66 in a red open-top classic Chevy, on the slow lane of the A14 in a grey SUV which scored solid marks across the board for safety and headroom? Is it always necessary to throw the TV out of the hotel window? Isn't 'leaving the room in the same condition in which you found it' just as much of a satisfying anecdote?

It's high time someone found out the answers to these burning questions. And seeing as it's my name on the front of this book,* I suppose it'll have to be me. But how did I come to be curious about such matters? I'll tell you. A handful of years ago I moved, with my then wife, Rhi, to a house on a quiet street in a quiet town and lay quietly in a room for a long time. I used to love an adventure, and I had jobs on magazines (remember magazines?) which provided the opportunity for plenty of them, but when I hit my thirties I started to become increasingly afraid of the world, until I was too frightened to even go outside. I'd been trying to keep fit and active by seeing a personal trainer a few times a week, but eventually I even sacked that off, giving myself completely to being isolated and horizontal. And I had no need to go outside: I'd somehow wangled it so that my job was mostly tweeting, which meant no colleagues, no bosses, no office, no alarm clock, no deadlines . . . just me, my phone and my social media feeds. Doesn't sound too healthy, does it? It wasn't. Everything went bad.

Eventually, slowly, with a lot of help, things started to become a little better. Once I'd been dragged out of the rooms I'd trapped myself in, I decided to try to make up for lost time. I wanted to be a bit less Pooh (Bear) and a bit more Grylls (Bear). I needed to set sail for 'Onwards!' – wherever that was – and unearth the dormant adventurer within. For a bit. For a whole year, in fact. I could do 50 adventures. That's a good number. Much less pleased with itself than 100. Perhaps I'd learn something about myself, such as:

---

* Hello!

- I can actually do lots of things and enjoy them
- I can't do anything without panicking and I'm better off not trying
- Some kind of middle ground between the above
- I've overreached myself with a fourth bullet point

To be honest, I had no idea what I was doing, I just knew I had to do something. Hopefully you'll have as much fun reading about my adventures* as I experienced going on them, i.e., 'a moderate amount of fun, at times'. Strap in,† then, please – it's gonna be a mild ride.

Rob

---

* Gentle attempts to find a hobby.
† Pithy joshing and pretty standard 'start of book banter' aside, please do always strap in when inside a moving vehicle. I know I'm not your mum, but it is for your own good, and it's also the law.

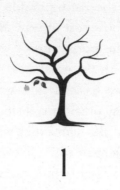

1

'Erm, I've got a room booked? Under the name Temple?'

'Mr . . . ah, Temple?'

'Yes, that's the one.'

I'm in Barcelona, where I know I've booked a room, so I'm not sure why I sound so suspicious of myself. Come to think of it, the lady on reception seems suspicious of me. Maybe I'm not Mr Temple, in which case . . . who am I? 'A-ha, yes, Temple. Robert, yes?' she says to the computer. That's me! I nod and we both allow ourselves a chuckle of relief: we've cracked the case, solved the puzzle. It's a curious game.

It's the first time I've left home for months. A particularly debilitating episode of ill health, the mental kind leading to the physical kind, has had me recuperating (or wallowing) safely (or dangerously) behind the curtains. If I'm going to reboot myself as an intrepid adventurer, the ability to travel solo seems mandatory; it's to adventuring what being able to carry a heavy bag is to army-ing. I've never really 'travelled'. I've been to a fair few places – from Tenby to Tokyo – but

I haven't travelled in the dating profile, gap year, beaded-bracelets-up-to-the-elbow sort of way. Nor have I travelled solo, apart from on the press trips of yonks ago, but then you always meet up with the usual crew of journos on those anyway. Press trips are basically just going to the pub by plane. So I've hurled my precious collection of caution to the wind and whooshed to Barcelona on a whim, despite generally being pretty deficient in whim. Now, sitting on the end of one of two tightly tucked twin hotel beds, shoes lined up under a desk, pants and socks in the most suitable drawers and passport in the safe, staring at my reflection in the black screen of the Philips telly, I'm hoping my whim replenishes itself enough to let me at least leave the room before it's time to fly home.

A few days earlier:

'Come and look at this,' says Mum. Mum says a lot of things to me these days, as does Dad, because I've recently moved back in with them. She's found another video of a cat on her iPad. She loves her iPad, and cats.

'Nah, it's okay, I'm not really interested,' I reply, immediately feeling disappointed in myself for not simply looking.

'You're not interested in anything.'

'I am!'

'Like what?'

'I ... I don't know. Jogging? I could always get back into jogging, I suppose. Bit cold, though. Or I could become a travelling man. Yes. I'll go travelling. On my own.'

'Are you sure that's a good idea?'

'Yes, I think I could become a travel man.'

'On your own?'

'Yeah.'

'Who with?'

'Just me, seeing the world, like Richard Ayoade in that *Travel Man* show.'

'Don't forget he's got a camera crew. And he goes with someone. And he gets paid for it.'

'I'll be fine.'

'So what will you do, while travelling?'

'Oh, loads of stuff. I'll take life by the horns.'

'Good. You be careful. Horns are dangerous.'

I'm thirty-five. It's about time I became interested in something, got some purpose and direction, instead of blindly bumbling around my life as if it's someone else's kitchen. I've taken to skulking through life, quietly puzzled, hesitant to make a fuss, an intern in my own existence. But what to do? There are so many things. The world is my oyster. I hate oysters. They make me sick.

Goa, Bali, Thailand ... They're all so far away. And expensive. And probably stuffed with the bracelet people. Where should I go? Where's good in January? I spin the globe and after a few attempts manage to make my finger land on Spain. Then, once it has, I manoeuvre the finger (index, of course, I'm not mad) deftly down to Barcelona. It's close enough to home, and I've been there many times. Good, I'll post myself there. Booking a last-minute ticket, I head straight out to buy a travel bag. Well, not straight out. I still have a few days until the departure date, I'm not going to book properly *last* minute, what with all the mini toiletries, airport parking/ route planning, insurance and other bits of admin I have to complete. I also have to visit Office World, as I'm fresh out of transparent plastic document wallets.

I also like to have a few days' cushion to decide whether I want to abort this, or any, idea or not. Present Me is always busy having to cancel all the stuff that Past Me thought would be fun to arrange. If I'm considering doing something wild and spontaneous, I make sure to thoroughly plan it out first. I visualise the whole scenario, summoning up as much negative energy as possible. If potential pros of the adventure outweigh the cons, which is rare, only then will I green-light the scheme; only then can I start worrying about it properly.

There's a few rucksacks and holdalls in TK Maxx, but they don't seem like they'd withstand a bashing should Ryanair decide I deserve the privilege of unexpectedly having my cabin bag chucked in the hold, like the last time I went on holiday (not that this is a holiday – this is travelling, I can't stress that enough). But it's my cabin bag, I'd argued, it has all my cabin stuff in it. 'But we're giving you access to the hold for free!' came the reply. There's nothing like the gift of being forced into a situation you don't want. There'd be no moisturising my face, cleaning my teeth, reading all five auto-biographies or changing my socks on that two-hour flight: those dreams were suffocating under the weight of other people's massive suitcases in the hold, and I was quietly livid. Also I'm doubtful these soft bags TK Maxx has a glut of meet Ryanair's regulations. Sure, one of these so-called 'travel' bags would fit the size-testing box thing in the airport if squished, but should it be full to capacity and therefore unsquishable, I'd be in trouble. The 30 cm shatterproof ruler I have with me is screaming, under the hot glare of the shop lights, 'DO NOT BUY THIS BAG!' So, despite the risk of not looking very traveller-y, I'm going for this smart, navy wheelie case made by Antler, complete with combination lock. Off to

Superdrug, then, just a few shops down in Huntingdon's 'big store' square, for my mini toiletries and . . . Ooh, what's this, a zip-up transparent toilet bag 'designed for flight'? Sold.

'Flying somewhere?' asks the man manning the till, who seems to have asked his tattooist for one of everything.

'Yes.'

'Nice one. I hate flying myself.' Get someone else to do it, then?

'Yeah, me too.'

'I'm always scared the plane's gonna burst into flames.'

'Right-o.'

My last stop is at Clifford's the Chemist in Godmanchester, just down the road from home, to pick up my thyroid medicine. I don't have a thyroid any more, so if I don't take pills I slowly swell up to the size of a mattress and then slip into a coma and die. This nearly happened at a wedding. I fell asleep in the corner of a pub for hours. The doctor told me that my body had gone into hibernation mode 'like a turtle', and it was a wonder I woke up. I should probably pick up some Pro Plus while I'm at the chemist, and mosquito spray, and some lip balm. And maybe some antihistamine. Plasters!

Ding-a-ling sounds the bell on the weathered white wooden door just off the mini-roundabout to the left of the Chinese Bridge. 'Be with you in a minute,' beams the pharmacist, as she rushes to the far shelf to pick up a packet of four toilet rolls. The room smells of lemon Lockets. 'I'm so sick of playing Russian roulette in that bloody toilet, I'm going to do something about it!' We both laugh conspiratorially and roll our eyes as she thumps off back up the stairs while I remain awkwardly rooted by the generous selection of plastic pillboxes. I have no idea what she means.

It's a couple of very early trains (I quickly decided against the hassle of driving/parking) to the airport. Huntingdon to Peterborough, Peterborough to Stansted. It's January-cold. I perch on the thin, freezing bench (on my arse, not like a canary) and tense everything, retracting into myself like a spooked whelk, while teenagers in school blazers chirp in sarcastic bursts and giggles around me. Peterborough station (the only conversation I ever hear about Peterborough involves the station: 'Oh yeah, I know Peterborough, I had to go to the station once') is full of folks on their way to the office, most of them looking like ticket collectors thanks to those black, baggy, strappy laptop bags. Boarding an end carriage of the empty Stansted train as the sun rises over the city – yes, it's a city: it has a cathedral! – I'm tremendously relieved to find my reserved aisle seat is available. Once I'm nestled in the plush but stained ruby-red bucket chair that looks like it's from a 1970s adult cinema, a round-headed fellow, a small face drawn in the dead centre of a taut balloon, who's holding a croissant and smells strongly of B&H, as if he's got a collection of half-smoked ones in his pocket, boards and, oh god, talks to me. He says he'd *prefer* to sit in my seat rather than in his assigned window seat. 'I've reserved this, I'm afraid. There are loads of free seats, though?' I say as I gesture to an empty carriage. 'Maybe if no one gets on later, I could sit in your seat?' he counters through his tiny little mouth, which is perfect for smoking. I'm stumped as to what kind of offer he thinks he's working with here, so I stay quiet. Eventually he goes away but leaves the smell of old tobacco behind, which is surprisingly quite comforting. The sky over Cambridgeshire glows red like Campari. Sight and smell and warmth combine, sending tingles up my neck. I feel an almost morphine-like wooziness wash through me. The first leg of a journey complete and out of my hands, I remain comfortably numb as the train slides me gently towards London. Not even the sight of Tobacco Man standing up to let a scatter of pastry flakes fall from his chest on to the floor manages to get my goat. Much.

Stansted is busy with travellers in dark coats and red scarves – apart from one lady in a dressing gown – spending their Christmas money, trudging wearily around like Lowry people. I wonder how I've been allowed, once again, to go through an airport unchaperoned, reminding myself that it's because I'm apparently an adult. In the queue for boarding, the chap in front of me, who looks just like a longer, thinner Iain Duncan Smith, is doing full-on running stretches for a good twenty minutes. His wild lunging really starts to irk me. Waiting until he's balancing on one leg, stretching out his quads, I consider giving him a gentle push, but then worry that I might get tasered. Christ, I'm knackered, drained from running on fake bravado all morning, from trying to walk with a sense of purpose; exhausted from attempting to not look constantly lost and through forcing myself to speak clearly and at a volume higher than my usual mumble. 'Bumbling Bernard' is one of my characters but it's not right for this situation. To get to the plane from the front door I have to be 'Confident Colin'. It's important to look like you have a clue what you're doing, to match everyone else doing the same.

'Flight 1234 is ready for boarding, please make your way to the departure gate.' All travellers on flight 1234 to Barcelona are already at the departure gate – we've been here for ages – but determined to respond to the instruction in some token way we stand a bit straighter, realign our rucksacks on our shoulders and shuffle forward an inch or two. *GO GO GO!* My brain is shouting at my heart to race and for my legs to shake, but the propranolol I took in Itsu keeps my body in neutral. I wish I'd taken it earlier for when security deemed my zip-up transparent toilet bag 'designed for flight' completely unsuitable for flight (cheers, Superdrug) and handed me a much smaller transparent bag that would help keep the plane in the sky. If every day is a school day, then today's lesson is that toothpaste will react to trying to be stuffed into something small and tight by ejaculating all over your arm.

I sit in my aisle seat and watch everyone file on with their wheelie cases the size of refrigerators and spend the flight staring open-mouthed at a snaggle-toothed, Einstein-haired man, clearly thirty to forty years away from being a child but nonetheless dressed like some sort of beach bum toddler, who considers it perfectly acceptable to read a book while idly digging into various bits of his head, before crumbling whatever he excavates between his fingers, casually seasoning the floor with his bodily waste. I dream of clicking his seat belt buckle mid-flight and opening the door. I dream this all the way to Spain, where I'm glad to be off the aircraft, which I feel should now be placed in a hospital toxic waste bin.

I hit the empty taxi rank at Barcelona airport. 'No taxi.' No taxi? 'No taxi.' So ... no taxi? Cab? 'No taxi.' It doesn't seem to matter how many times I have it confirmed there are no taxis, the taxi situation simply refuses to resolve. Finally the penny drops: no taxis! Right, time to move directly to the fifth stage of grief and accept that I have to find a train or, good lord, a sodding bus into the city. Breathe. I am Columbus. After studying the train map for about half an hour, I deduce that every train which leaves Barcelona El Prat Airport appears to just go somewhere into the middle of the main bit, which is roughly where my hotel lives, so I hop on one of them and hop off half an hour later at Passeig de Gràcia, walking a further half an hour in the Catalan winter sunshine. Phone now switched to 'Movistar', I Instagram a few things along the way – a road sign, my own face in sunglasses, a fountain – to persuade people I'm happy, and amble past swarms of on-strike black and yellow cabs, colossal metal bumblebees in search of a giant peach, to the Hotel Universal.

It's a very plain hotel. The type of place you go for a conference. I thought about getting a B&B, but every time I do that I seem to end up becoming part of a family for the duration of my stay. A trip to Norfolk had the husband explaining to me that his wife likes to stay in a dark room watching tennis all day (never saw her), so I was welcome to hang out with him. I didn't actually see much of him in the end, as he kept having to 'pop to the woods'. Just outside the main door of the hotel, a man with an Irish accent asks to borrow my phone. 'I was DJing up in the mountains and now I have to call me mother.' It's not the most convincing story I've heard. 'I'm really sorry, I can't give you my phone,' I reply. 'I'm going in this door now, sorry.' He tells me to piss off (which is surely what I'm already doing?) and to go and have sex with myself (on my list). There was a kid at my school who at the age of eight swore blind he invented the insult 'piss off'. Mad to think it's made it all the way to Barcelona. Anyway, I'm here, with my little suitcase, I have arrived. 'Erm ... I have a room booked?'

'Coke, hash, blow job?' I'm asked by a young brunette lady in black high heels, tight blue jeans and an oversized pink puffa jacket as I'm on my way, layered up against the chill, down the dark Gothic Quarter streets off La Rambla for dinner at a restaurant that specialises in snails. I've been holding myself hostage in the hotel for a day and a night and another day, only letting myself out once to go to the supermarket next door. I used up so much energy summoning the gall to leave the safety of my room to journey to the solitary safety of another room, that I'm now spent. Life would be fine if it was just going from room to room. The outside world, with all its people and wide open space, really does throw a spanner in the works. Coke, hash, blow job? Certainly not in that order, I think, hurrying head down past the bright mobile phone shops of Carrer dels Escudellers. No, that just personally wouldn't be workable.

I first came to Los Caracoles with my partner at the time, Gemma, about ten years ago, but we had to leave because fish soup, a big plate of monstrous boiled slugs (not the French garlicky morsels – these were nightmarish giant snot creatures) and a vicious hangover had me feeling delirious and sweaty, my mind as wonky as a Dalí clock. You enter the place through a door (classic) into a bar, which you walk through into the kitchen, which leads into a reception area, then through to ever-deepening caves of dining rooms. You stop at each leg of this journey to say to someone, anyone, 'I have a reservation?' This person then seems completely shocked/put out to see a customer or to have it suggested that the place is even a public eating establishment at all. It's as if you're walking into a series of strangers' living rooms and asking for supper. It also seems to be a rule here that every waiter be a cross bald man. Some online reviewers have typed their opinion that it's a tourist trap. I knew all this, but after spending a day online looking for a hip new joint in which to feast on the latest in Catalan cuisine, alone, I became paralysed by choice. The waiter takes my order, not looking at me, my menu or even his own pad as he writes, but instead gazing angrily across the room like he's having a flashback to a nightmarish childhood trip to the seaside. I feel on edge, unable to get warm; I'm stiff-necked and stranded. One small sip of wine would melt all the unease away.

'Yes?'

'Erm ... I'll have,' I panic, '... the fish soup.'

'Yes?'

'Oh. More? Okay, I'll have some fries as well. *Fritas*?'

'Yes?'

'That's it.'

'That's it?'

'That's it.'

'One soup, one *fritas*.'

'Yes, please.'

'Nothing else?'

'Just another Coke would be great.'

He whisks the wine glasses away as if they've answered him back once too many times and he now intends to give them a damn good thrashing once he's alone with the pair of clinky bastards.

The soup, rich with shell juice, is the type of curry powder/ turmeric colour that really stains white linen when splashed about by a shaky man's spoon. Soon the tablecloth looks like someone's shot the yellow Teletubby in the back of the head over it. The soup costs more than this specific soup should. The *fritas* never arrived. Time to scurry away, bedways is rightways, as they say in *A Clockwork Orange*, though I'm sure they got that from my Mum.

My supermarket trip has provided me with Milka chocolate, which I kept in my mind throughout the meal as something to look forward to, a ton of gummy sweets, paprika crisps, two bottles of water, a new mini toothpaste and a block of hard white vacuum-packed cheese that I keep in the minibar fridge perched atop two cans of Estrella, and which I later open most horrifyingly with mini toenail clippers.

My only other meal 'out' is in the hotel restaurant, a short ride up in the lift. The Wolf Tavern doesn't know if it wants to be an Italian deli, a British pub, an American diner or a sports bar, so it combines elements of all of them to create a weird whole that's none of them. It's already half set up for breakfast in the morning, which is a bit depressing. I feel more self-conscious than usual, as back in my room I mistook my toothpaste for lip balm and smeared Colgate all over my mouth; now I'm having my doubts as to whether I got it all off.

'Are you ready perhaps for something to eat?'

'Yes please, is it okay to order a chicken Caesar salad, but is it also okay to have some croquettes on the side?'

'Salad and croquettes.'

'If that's okay?'

'Anything else?'

'No, *gracias*.'

A lower-division Spanish football match plays on one of the large tellies, which gives me something to stare at, although I don't hear the match because the tellies are all on mute while Shania Twain's 'Man! I Feel Like A Woman' plays through loudspeakers. And technically I don't even really watch the match, I just stare in its general direction and pretend to watch, meaning I'll eat my meal with my head turned 90 degrees to the left, so that anyone else who might enter the otherwise empty room won't think I'm just there to do something as deviant as eat alone at 7 p.m.; no, I'm here for the sport, thank you. I'm annoyed with myself: why can't I just relax and have a laugh? I used to have a lot of laughs; now I just feel like I'm constantly killing time. It would be easier if I was pissed. Yay – my salad is being carried towards me! Time to sit up a bit more and re-straighten my knife and fork, then move them outwards a bit more so the plate doesn't accidentally clank on them. I straighten a tie that isn't there, flatten my shirt over my belly and prepare to say, 'That's lovely, thank you, great stuff, *gracias.*' The salad is in some kind of black plant pot, with KFC-style fried popcorn chicken, iceberg lettuce that seems to have been fed through a paper shredder and the dressing in an artful Z shape across the top, as if, with a flourish, Zorro has jizzed on my meal. *Olé!* Why is hotel food so weird? Trying to please everyone, I suppose.

The table next to me fills up with five suits, who start discussing business in the hope of pleasing someone called Roger, who's apparently not happy. Now all I can do is listen to them. There must be over thirty tables in here, and they choose the one next to me. One of their satchels is touching my thigh, and a man with stubble you could sand a bench on is eyeing up my croquettes while rubbing his bicep. Maybe if I give him a stare ... Nope, that was a bad idea. Couldn't commit to it, ended up turning it into a smile. Quick, look to the ceiling. Look everywhere and smile! You're just a smiley guy, enjoying the ambience. I must look bonkers. What am I doing? This is just awful. I must leave. I feel like I might faint. Are my hands going blue? I think my hands might be turning blue.

I ask if I can take the croquettes back to my room (party time!) as if requesting nuclear codes. 'Of course,' says the waitress, of course, and I scuttle away with my little cellophaned side plate and get in bed fully clothed. I shouldn't have come here. I don't sleep well during my stay because it's chilly in the room. I know there are extra blankets in the wardrobe, I've seen them, but I never quite manage to give myself the push to get up and unfold them. Instead I lie there for half the night, just a tiny bit too cold for comfort, thinking about getting the blankets. This sort of thing has always been a problem. I let small things build, until they form a stack that feels unmanageable. I allow bills to pile. I live for years with computer viruses, working my way around them with an ever-diminishing array of workable computer functions at my disposal. If a letter disappeared from my keyboard, I'd use words that don't rely on it. I survived a whole year with a laptop that insisted on speaking French. Some of it is laziness, mixed with the illogical belief that if I don't do anything then nothing can go wrong. Also mixed into the concoction that makes up my uselessness is an ever-present urge to self-sabotage. Historically, as soon as life seems to be trundling along quite harmlessly, I'll try to make it all a bit more exciting. I'll try to make a change to spice things up a bit, and that change will almost without exception be rash, ill-thought-out, against all sensible advice and not at all conducive to maintaining a healthy mental outlook.

I get trapped in hotel rooms. I'm ready to leave two hours before checkout, in this instance heavily sugared up with Fruittella, but I'm unable to exit a room unless it's bang on the deadline, which isn't helpful for the cleaners. I'm worrying about how I've been too scared to make this trip interesting.

Miles: 1,000, anecdotes: nil. Outside is all the world: a stage, apparently. And I'm here, frozen in the wings.

'Can we get you a taxi?' asks the receptionist.

'No thank you, I'll be fine!'

It takes me half an hour of wandering back alleys before I locate a cab. My remaining euros go towards a Barcelona FC pencil case from the airport, for my nephew James, which I study while sat in a restaurant. *JAMON! JAMON JAMON JAMON!* shouts the laminated A4 poster taped to the wall. The place is full of happy couples sipping mini bottles of screw-top cava. Actually, only one couple is doing that, but loudly. Have you ever looked directly upwards while sat in an airport pub or café? It's all steel beams and girders and corrugated roofing. Feels like you're on a film set. I'm waiting for the director to shout 'Action!' so I can get my small part over with. My flight is called and I journey home – my first adventure in the bag/wheelie case – with few tales to tell.

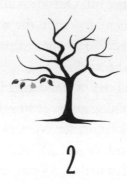

2

It's not until you have a desire to do yoga that you notice just how much the country's stuffed with it. Every other building in the UK has people of all shapes and ages in Lycra, bending themselves silly and trying not to parp. And we're all destined to do it at least once. It's the jury duty of exercise. My time has come; I've summoned myself.

Why yoga? Well, you see, I've always wanted to be a zen guy. As a young teen I used my pocket money to buy peace symbol necklaces on family holidays. I had a best of Bob Marley CD. I painted my bedroom brown and burned incense. I even attempted to smoke incense through a pipe, which burned my throat terribly, though not as savagely as the cinnamon stick, or the 'purple haze' legal high my friend Jas and I smoked on a wall in our school uniforms, an old lady calling us naughty boys as the loosely rolled joint went up in flames like dry hay (probably what it was) and disappeared our fluffy moustaches, which at the time really harshed our vibes. 'Scuse me while I miss the sky. I'd like to recapture those hippy aspirations, in a healthier, less stupid way.

Where to find yoga round here? This requires the help of the splendid Godmanchester Living Facebook page. I'm addicted to it. Nothing shows the strengths, gripes, heart and hilariousness of a town like the community Facebook page. It's a digital town hall where everyone's invited. A place where the town's residents rush to say they've stepped in dog mess, or to offer someone a lift to the hospital, or to thank someone for helping them park; to say someone shifty's going round in a van, or to ask about the A14, or to state that a delivery driver has thrown their parcel in a pond, or occasionally just to say something a little bit uncomfortable. My favourite posts recently have been about 1. A turtle that keeps escaping, and 2. A friendly seal who lives in the nature reserve, though not everyone was delighted with the seal's presence – 'He'll eat all the fish!' Another personal favourite: 'Is this anyone's chicken?' Godmanchester Living finds me a weekly evening yoga group in the neighbouring village of Hartford, which I often drive through en route to the nearest twenty-four-hour Big Tesco, and I pay for six beginner sessions.

The initial instructions advise against trying to access the building via a certain long, thin lane, so I do exactly this, eventually having to reverse all the way back. Extracting myself backwards down this muddy track without destroying my car is more tense than a game of Operation. The printout also advises me not to drive too far into the car park in the dark, else there's a high chance I'll go straight into the river. It's a stressful journey. I'll need some yoga by the time I arrive. Turning off my engine, thankfully with no water around the pedals, I'm just in time to witness an odd exchange between two women in gym kits who I assume are here for the same reason as I am.

'Do you want me to guide you in?' says the helpful lady in the already parked shiny white 4 × 4. She's prim and manicured, in her fifties, perhaps, looking as if she's journeyed out for a posh lunch but has capriciously veered right to a random church hall in the hope of a good old stretching.

'No, I was a driving instructor for ten years,' comes the curious and curt reply from the less glam, no-nonsense woman with hair like mine, in the hatchback, who does some kind of six-point manoeuvre to reverse-park into a random area of this large square of empty nothing. There aren't any bays or lines, just ground. Perhaps she can see some markings that the rest of us can't; I mean, she had been a driving instructor for ten years, a fact she repeats a further two times before we get into the building, then twice more once we do. 'I said to her, I said I'd been a driving instructor for ten years, love, I don't need help parking . . . Oh, hello love, sorry, I didn't mean to be rude out there, it's just that I used to be a driving instructor, so I'm quite used to parking . . .' If she was my driving instructor, not only would I know it, but I'd make damn sure I passed my test first time. I wouldn't want to disappoint her.

Everyone else has mats under their arms, I notice. And towels. I feel quite naked just standing here in my running kit and bright red flip-flops. I'm nervous, and concentrate on smiling politely and chuckling whenever anybody (all older women) says anything. Bloody hell, I'm shaking. They all speak entirely in jokey complaints, the punchlines of which seem to consist solely of eye-rolls and saying, 'I don't know, eh?' I hand over my payment to the instructor, Emmi, with shaky hands, like I'm paying for drugs ... *Got any downward dog?* She lends me a mat. We spread ourselves out, as instructed, our mats our little personal islands in the sea, and spend the next hour desperately trying not to accidentally look at anyone else's arse, which is tricky when you're surrounded by them.

Emmi's really chilled, as you'd expect, I suppose – it'd be worrying to have a really uptight yoga instructor – and makes us comfortable and encourages us to move at our own pace, wobbly and slow being the most favoured speed. She looks like she does a lot of yoga: that is, toned, bendy and possessing of a peaceful aura. I bought my gym kit a few years ago to grow into, which I've done rather too enthusiastically, especially since I gave up on personal training last year. I'm like dough wrapped in cling film, proving in a cupboard. I start to do some casual stretches, in preparation for the hour-long casual stretchathon about to commence, though I think I might be wrong to do so. But as Emmi says, there is no wrong way to do things here. I like it when someone says that. It makes me want to push the good faith implied in the statement to the limit; to fire up Netflix on my phone and get out a ham sandwich in the middle of the session. This is because I'm childish. 'Sorry I'm late, traffic was terrible,' says the harassed lady who bustles in late. 'That's okay, just grab a space, you haven't missed much at all,' says Emmi, peacefully. 'I got stuck on that bloody ring road, just before the turn-off ...' Harassed Lady continues, hoovering up any burgeoning bits of zen with every word. I smile three or four times when I think she's about to look at me, but each time it's a false alarm. I'm shaking even more now. Still ages to go. Time is taking forever.

There are six or seven of us, the largest class Emmi has taught so far. On one side of the hall, which smells faintly of hymn books, sweat and coffee breath – all church halls smell the same, a smell I can only term, perhaps owing to a disappointing vocabulary, as a bit 'churchy' – is a big window looking out on to a graveyard. 'Just ignore them,' Emmi says, as we turn to face the rows of stones. Ignore them? Maybe we could learn from them. Can't get more relaxed than them, really. In many ways, they've reached peak yoga.

There are so many joints popping in the room it sounds like we're going gung-ho with a box of Christmas crackers. Despite the plinky-plonky hippy chill-out coming from the chubby little portable plastic CD player, the grey type with the flimsy carry handle and random bits of neon blue, the atmosphere in the room isn't overly relaxed, if I'm honest. But then we are all beginners. The lady next to me keeps doing the rolling-her-eyes-and-tutting thing, which I do back to her, as if we're asking each other, 'What's all this about, eh? What are we doing here?' and the woman who used to be a driving instructor keeps stating that she can't do yoga because of her sciatica. 'If there are any parts that make you feel uncomfortable or that you don't want to try, that's absolutely fine,' Emmi gently stresses, prompting a long response about troublesome elbows. My back hurts and my legs seem to be made of jelly. I nearly had a stroke trying on some skinny jeans in a Big Tesco fitting room the other day (at least, I think they were skinny jeans – perhaps they were regular jeans and I have fatty thighs). This feels a bit like that. The main sounds in the room, other than cracking, are *oof!* and *bloody 'ell!* I've gone all light-headed. I'm greying out! I need a lie-down. Hang on, I *am* lying down. Yoga, or at least my attempt at yoga, has managed to make lying down – my favourite thing! – seem difficult. Everyone starts having a conversation about how the class is at an inconvenient time, as if it's compulsory community service yoga – 'I'll have to have my dinner at 9 p.m., I only finished work an hour ago' – before someone's car alarm goes off for the remaining half an hour. 'Sorry, I think that might be mine,' says the woman who belongs to the arse in front of me. Although she doesn't check if it definitely is indeed her BMW that's wailing through the wall.

'How's everyone feeling?' Emmi asks, receiving the awkward and inevitable response of complete silence. 'That's excellent.' I'm feeling white and weak, like I've simultaneously lost all my blood sugar and had ten espressos. After five minutes of pretending to sleep, I gather my things, wave goodbye to the room and speed out the door as if late for an important meeting. Leaving the car park, I pull out straight into a traffic jam. The radio keeps switching itself on and off and I look at my watch while holding a half-full can, resulting in warm, flat Diet Coke spilling over my crotch. Good.

'I don't think I'm built for yoga,' I tell my parents while getting some crisps from the cupboard.

'Stop eating crisps!' shouts Mum. 'You won't get slim eating crisps! Anyway, tea'll be ready soon.'

'What we having?'

'I don't know,' replies Mum, 'depends on what you're making. What's that on your shorts? Looks like you've wet yourself.'

'I could get sausage and mash from the Co-op?'

'Yes, that'd be nice. Dad likes that. Don't forget to buy gravy. You like that, don't you, Paul?'

'What's that?'

'Sausages and mash, you like that, don't you?'

'Yes, lovely, I like anything.'

'Right-o,' I say, scrubbing myself with a baby wipe, which makes matters damper. 'Any sausage preference?'

'Ooh, I quite like those Colombian ones!'

Mum's stumped me with this one. I work out in the Co-op that she must mean Cumbrian. It's a good job she's not a drug baron, ordering fifty kilos of finest Cumbrian cocaine.

'Just these, please, mate,' I say to the young chap at the counter. 'How are you doing today?'

'I'm alive and kicking, thank you, sir, can't ask for more than that!'

'I suppose not.'

As I fork mash into my mouth, I wonder ... perhaps I'm just too het up to ever be zen. Perhaps I don't try hard enough. Trying to be zen seems like an oxymoron, but I suppose even relaxing takes work. I used to seek out extreme challenges. Ultramarathons, that sort of caper. That year or two of endless jogging, nearly a decade ago, was I think the most relaxed and happy I've been, but it was a bit unsustainable, mostly for my knees. Maybe yoga is too relaxing to relax me. As I squeeze some more ketchup on to the edge of my plate, on top of the HP, English mustard and chilli sauce that's already there (I love a condiment), I think that maybe I need to suffer over a fifty-mile jog with blood seeping from my nipples to feel truly chilled.

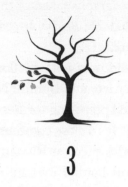

3

Home is Godmanchester – that place I've already mentioned a few times which, unless you're from Godmanchester, has made you think, 'What in the name of hell is a Godmanchester? Is it like a Wonderwall? Is it a superior Manchester?' No. Godmanchester is a pretty town in Cambridgeshire. It's like the setting for a gentle children's cartoon, full of shopkeepers and postmen.

You could have a wonderful life here. It has four pubs – The White Hart, The Royal Oak, The Exhibition, which is next to the house with the tree that spills figs on Earning Street, and The Black Bull – a few cafés and two Co-ops. There's a family-run butcher's, a fishing tackle and trophy-engraving shop, a riverside chippy where the owner at the time angrily threw a saveloy at my head, Bellmans the sandwich place, a couple of newsagents, an Indian restaurant called Planet Spice and a Chinese restaurant called Cinta; ducks, geese and swans, Union Jack bunting in summer, a big Christmas tree in winter and the Chinese Bridge that appears in about

95 per cent of all photographs taken of the place. The town's own magazine is called *The Bridge*. It often has a picture of the bridge on the cover.

Godmanchester loves occasions. Halloween is a big thing here, as is the summer fete and Bonfire Night. The community has already started preparing for Remembrance Sunday and it's only February. It's a close community, really. A small one. I once stood in the queue at Roman Gate, the surgery, and my neighbour was behind me and my sister-in-law in front. 'What are you here for, then?' 'Oh, just ill, you know,' I said as I slid my scrap of paper with *ANXIETY* written on it in shaky letters to the receptionist. It's twenty minutes to Cambridge by car and an hour to King's Cross by rail from the adjoining larger town of Huntingdon.

Rhi and I met at the gadget magazine we worked at ten years ago, marrying four years later, and set up home in Balham. Five years ago we bought a house in Godmanchester to try to start a family with a bit of affordable space. Now I live temporarily with my parents, just down the road. I say temporarily; it's been about a year. Or maybe two now? I can't remember, every day is the same. I remember I was living by myself in February 2018, which was when my mental health really took a nosedive, during the Beast from the East which covered the country in thick snow. After that, for a while, my own sense of time became unreliable.

It's very peaceful at Mum and Dad's. They have a wonderful apple tree that creates enough crumble to last all winter. We're only halfway through the last batch. Some people struggle to move back in with their parents, but I've perhaps found it a bit too comforting for my own good. Mum and Dad are very zen, but then they have quite a set routine which they don't enjoy deviating from. They maintain their zen with rigorous planning. A lot of training and rules seem to go into being relaxed. They've given me stability when I had become a train so far off the rails I was upside down in a cow field, and I'll always be grateful for it. Plus, while I'm here I can help with cooking, shopping and heavy lifting, so I think they're as happy with the current deal as I am.

I've driven to our house, or 'the marital home' as solicitors call it, to check for post, most of which is addressed to Mr Pizza Lover. No matter how long the house sits cold and empty, and how much multipurpose Flash is sprayed, it still smells of last year's life, now as dead as the chilli plants in the garden. It smells of Raffy, our Bernese Mountain Dog, who died at two from a spinal stroke. I don't like to stay in this house for too long. It's the scene of a breakdown. Memories collide with the dust, catching in my eyes and throat like pollen. Clutching my wedge of takeaway menus, which I'll enjoy reading later, I look at the grey sofa – everything in this house is grey, or 'Elephant Dung' or 'Weimaraner Sigh' or whatever it was we picked.

The last time I was sat on that sofa, a few days after my old friend Andy (we bonded at school over both trying to be hippies) had visited and cleaned the place up, taking out all the empties and clearing up the smashed glass and overflowing bins and cooked me some pasta, I felt so glum and done in that my chest started to physically hurt, like I was being repeatedly stabbed with a rusty tent peg. It turned out to be acute pancreatitis. If you've never had it I wouldn't bother, if I were you. It really, really hurts. Imagine someone trying to remove the contents of your torso using only a rock and a shard of glass. If you did wish to get it, the quickest way that I know is to subsist on a diet of vodka and wine gums for a few months. My older brother Mark, a furniture designer who lives down the road with his wife Jane and little boy James and teenage daughter-in-law Emily who he met when he met Jane, drove me and my yellow eyes to Hinchingbrooke hospital. Once speedily admitted into A&E, then just as speedily into a ward, my mind fully disintegrated. I hallucinated that I was in a prisoner-of-war camp, convinced that the pouch of piss attached to my leg was a bomb set to detonate at any moment. I barricaded myself in Bay Tree Ward bathroom and called the police for 'backup'. At one point I woke to see my family around my bed. My parents had been called back from their holiday in Spain. I nearly died, and when I didn't, I realised I didn't want to. Not for a while, anyway.

Now I'm outside my house, back in my car, looking up at the spare bedroom window. All the time, and not just my own time, I wasted behind that window . . . I just couldn't leave that house, not for years. 'You idiot,' I say to myself, 'why didn't you get hel—' Suddenly, WHAM! My phone's Bluetooth connects to the car stereo and blares 'Club Tropicana' in my face. It's impossible to be self-pitying when George Michael is singing to you about fun and sunshine. This year will not be wasted, even if it kills me. With solo travel (sort of) and yoga ticked off, I have forty-eight adventures to go.

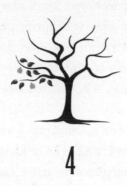

4

I've always wanted to know how to haggle. I'm simply no good when it comes to business. I've no nose for a deal. Unlike Dad, a retired accountant who once owned and ran the largest accountancy firm in Peterborough, I'm not a numbers guy. I've only ever paid full asking price, and sometimes more. I even paid for the non-existent *fritas* in Barcelona. What a mug. Haggling would make a fine adventure as well as coming in handy if I'm ever presented with the opportunity to purchase a large rug, possibly in Morocco. I've never been to Morocco. Always looks quite dusty on telly.

I'm thinking about this while sat in The Little Hair Boutique in St Ives (the Cambridgeshire one) having, unsurprisingly, a haircut. It's only a Tuesday morning in January but the sun's shining more like a Saturday lunchtime in March. The Little Hair Boutique is precisely named: a charming, bijou room with three chairs, tucked down a mews which is home to various other grooming parlours and the Rockabilly sandwich shop. St Ives, and Cambridgeshire in general, appears to me to have a lot of hair salons. My mum's salon in the 1960s, in nearby Whittlesey, was called Nova, which I think is pretty hip. She sold Avon products from there, which she wasn't technically allowed to do, so from inside the 'Nova' sign on the glass read backwards, revealing her dark secret.

I planned to ask for something 'completely different'. Something new and exciting. 'Go wild, shave half of it off, paint the other half purple, then shave that off, too,' I could say. After having my hair washed (I answer that the water temperature is fine, and luckily it is), and spending a couple of minutes fighting against the pleasant feeling of the head massage, Lisa, who runs The Little Hair Boutique, guides me freshly towelled into a chair and foot-pumps me upwards a few notches.

'So, what is it today?'

'Just a tidy-up, please. Shear off the grey.' I'm such a coward.

'It's blade three around the edges, isn't it?'

'Can we go for blade four this time?'

'Blade four, no problem. And you have it combed to the right, don't you?'

I consider changing things up and saying I want my fringe pointing left, but I worry this might permanently damage my parting, so just say 'yep'. We chat about the imminence of the clocks going back and Mother's Day, and then I feel guilty for letting my detached hair fall on the floor as I stand. I do enjoy having my hair cut, though, despite all the mini awkwardnesses. The awkwardness of haircuts has a lot to answer for: my first Very British Problems tweet, back in 2012, was about trying to pull off a slightly shorter haircut than normal. I wish hair grew more quickly so I could have it cut more often; it's probably my favourite and most consistently practised social hobby.

I should probably explain what Very British Problems is. Back in 2012, one of my editors at the gadget magazine, Matt, suggested I should really have a Twitter account, being a tech journo and that. At the same time, my mate James sent me a list of twenty or so funny, clichéd things British people do. They were basically awkward situations … my speciality! 'Oh, there's far more than twenty,' I thought, so I set up a Twitter account – @SoVeryBritish – and started to tweet the various embarrassing situations I find myself in on a daily basis. Within a month I had 100,000 followers and I was contacted by Juliet, my literary agent, asking if we should make a book. I was living in Balham with Rhi at the time. As we were doing Dry January, we celebrated with champagne flutes of fizzy water.

Before long there were auctions, meetings and decisions. Then I was sat on a sofa facing some Skips and pork pies, part of a British picnic theme (though I don't remember eating anything; my mouth had completely dried up, so attempting a Skip – arguably the most dissolvable crisp – would have been like chewing a ball of paper), and talking to Hannah Boursnell, an editor of non-fiction at the Little, Brown publishing house.

Juliet did most/all of the talking, I did the shaking. Juliet is like a protective sister. She's one of the top agents in the country, delightful company, and looks after her writers fiercely and calmly. I bet, if needs be, she's able to hurl throwing stars to pin people to walls, but just doesn't talk about it. Think Hit-Girl, but grown up, more temper control and into books. Footnote: I asked Juliet yesterday if she actually had throwing stars in her desk. She wouldn't deny it.

Not that Hannah is in any way intimidating or needs protecting from; she's one of the friendliest people you could meet, but my brain is irrational and I could hardly talk in the meeting, or at least that's how I recall it, even though I'd dressed up all smart and had a notebook full of questions.

Then I wrote a book, *Very British Problems: Making Life Awkward for Ourselves, One Rainy Day at a Time*, and it was released, and people bought it. I was even invited to go and see the book printed. Literally hot off the presses! I felt a bit undeserving of such a privilege, but Juliet, Hannah and I boarded a train from Liverpool Street and made our way to the factory. I think someone was in our reserved seats, or we were in theirs. Anyway, it was all good material.

My most vivid memory of the occasion was being in a small room full of ink. I nearly collapsed with the strength of it. It was like entering a room full of loose petrol. Still, it was the ink that was creating a book with my name on it. It felt bizarre, watching pages of my words zipping by on big machines.

And people bought the thing. Celebrities commented nicely on it. I was invited on the radio to talk about it, and also on the telly (said no). Slowly I crept on to a whole new level of anxiety, brought about by attention. When you have a small panic attack when you think someone's staring at you in a supermarket, being tweeted at by strangers saying they thought you came across as boring on the radio, gives you a new level of the willies. Even though you know it's meaningless and 'running popular social media feed' is incredibly low-tier in the celeb scheme of things (is there a letter below Z?).

Now there are over five million followers, more books, board games, telly shows, merch, calendars ... and I get to work from my sofa. It's certainly been a strange and unexpected career trajectory.

Leaving the salon, after trying to wave to three different stylists using one big, ungainly wave, with newly chilly ears and the hairstyle I've had for the past fifteen years, I stroll out of Cromwell Mews, redo my hair in Stephens Butchers and Delicatessen window (why trust the professional who had a 360-degree view of my head to style it suitably?) and cross the road to the Hyperion Antiques Centre. Being freelance, I've watched a lot of *Cash in the Attic* and *Flog It!*. I also occasionally catch *Antiques Roadshow*, for that tangible back-to-school-tomorrow punch to the gut. There's no 'weekend is over' siren quite like watching someone having an old vase valued. Working mainly on social media, for myself, I don't have a nine-to-five week, so Sunday doesn't really mean anything, but I still get that 'work tomorrow' feeling of doom. I panic that I haven't done my homework. Sadly I don't still get the TGI Friday feeling; I used to love that.

I steady myself by a bench and take a deep breath. I am about to buy an antique/old bit of tat, to test if I have the ability to haggle. This adventure will not only take me out of my comfort zone, it has the potential to be beneficial to my life. There's a quirkier antique-y, vintage-y type shop in Huntingdon: Cambs Lock. I think it might even be quite famous. It's a vast warehouse of sprawling rooms of stuff. Big old-world hanging maps, gas masks (maybe I'll get one for Halloween), RAF outfits, 1950s Coke adverts, cigarette cards, glass paperweights, kooky chairs, toys, dolls, games, dice, penknives, typewriters, wooden chickens, kettles, bottle caps ... a lot of kitsch stuff. It looks like somewhere that could be raided to decorate every pub in Zone 2. But the Hyperion is a bit easier to navigate, and, well, it's right outside the hairdresser's.

The sign in the window says it opens at 9.30 a.m. I try the brass handle of the green door at 9.40 a.m. to find it locked. This startles the chap inside, dressed head to socks in English mustard yellow, who looks at his watch, shakes his head at himself and comes rushing with keys to unlock and let me in.

'Sorry!' I blurt.

'No, no, sorry, I was miles away, come in, haha.'

'Haha, sorry, thank you, sorry, I wasn't sure when you opened,' I lie.

'Haha, yes, yes.'

'Haha, anyway, good morning, thanks, haha.'

'Haha, yes ... yes ...'

It's unfortunate that we both have the exact same style of communication: fill any potential silence with forced chuckling until we pass away and finally relax. I've spent a hell of a lot of time laughing politely. I'm always trying to stop doing it, it's no good for anyone, but it just comes out. Being positive doesn't come naturally to me, I have to constantly learn how to do it from others; fake positivity, on the other hand, I'm well versed in. I wish I could just be a proper misery guts, one who really goes for it. The type of curmudgeon where people would say, 'Oh, don't mind him, you'll get used to it!', the grump who knows their act is creating amusement, and who has the strength of character to see it through. Fletcher in *Porridge* type of thing, instead of a shy, chuckling odd bod. Very rarely I'll encounter the type who responds to my chuckling with a confused, stern look. On one occasion someone even said, 'What's funny?' Yes! Indeed! What *is* funny?! Thank you for breaking the spell, now please punch me in the face. There's ego in all the forced chuckling; in bestowing a grin on someone. It's nerves and social incompetence, but also demonstrates a lack of trust that the person is capable of engaging with you in any sort of proper conversation. Of course, when I actually really need to laugh I hold it back with all my might, like Dad does, ending up looking like I'm desperately trying not to sneeze.

I slip away to start exploring this one-room, low-ceilinged bunker. A muzak version of 'What A Wonderful World' plays from somewhere, reminding me of my grandad, the late, great Louis Armstrong. Not really; my grandad was called Thomas and just liked that song. We played it at his funeral. The room smells how I imagine a headmaster's office would do in 1910 – a mixture of old paper and dressing-up box. The dust swirls and curls through the sunbeams and I have a strong desire to put on a military jacket and smoke a pipe while listening to county cricket on the wireless.

I stroll slowly and regally, weaving my way across the rough brown carpet, bits of hair falling from my shoulders, making sure to stop and pretend to admire something now and then. I imagine I'm Prince Charles judging a vegetable competition in a marquee in the Cotswolds. I even place my hands behind my back like a pro. What to buy? Maybe this rather grand velvet top hat? Or this fire poker that looks like a sword? Perhaps this splendid framed Miró print? A-ha, no, I see what I want; I clock what I must have; I discover what I need. My gaze is powerfully drawn towards an olive-green vase, or is it a jug? There's no handle to speak of, so I'll call it a vase. It has a face on it, resembling both the mask in the film *The Mask* and one of the talking trees in *The Lord of the Rings*. At the top is the word 'celery'. Yes, I think, this is it.

THIS IS IT! I am the beholder with an eye that thinks this item is beautiful. Demented, sure, but beautiful nonetheless. The little cardboard tag fastened with brown string says in scribbled blue biro: '16'. I walk it carefully to the till, past the silverware and decorative plates, a piano version of 'Bridge Over Troubled Water' playing in the glittery air, and say the words, 'Hello there, haha, I don't suppose you would part with this for . . . ten pounds?' Would you part with this?! Who do I think I am? Lovejoy? I feel nauseous.

'Oh, haha, no, I'm afraid not, haha.'

'Oh, okay.' Well, this isn't like on the telly.

'No discounts on anything under twenty pounds, I'm afraid.'

'Could you do anything with the price?'

'Haha, no, no.'

'It's just, I only have ten pounds in cash.'

'We take cards.'

'Oh . . . *oh*! Oh well then, that's perfect. Excellent. Sorry. Thank you!' I stand there, feeling like I've been caught trying to steal a . . . well, a celery jar. I burn with guilt.

'Okay, so that's sixteen pounds.'

'And you couldn't go to fifteen?' This is desperate stuff.

'Haha, no, no. Just pop your pin in, please.'

'Right you are.'

I leave the shop, apologising, with my £16 celery vase bubble-wrapped and brown-paper-bagged, stop in at Waitrose to buy my mum and dad some of the tartare sauce they like, and then sit peacefully in the car for a few minutes to regain my composure. I feel pretty good now, actually. That was fun. It was over quickly, didn't involve many people . . . would recommend. It's so perfectly warm in the car, I could fall asleep (I think I might secretly be a cat). At least I didn't insist on shaking hands while saying, 'Call it twelve and I'll take it away now.' Has anyone ever alternatively said, 'Tell you what, shake hands now and I'll leave the item with you for a fortnight'? What was I doing, trying to haggle for something under twenty quid anyway? The chap's gotta make a living, he can't just be giving his celery jars away. He's not a celery eater charity. On the way home I divert to Big Tesco to purchase the celery and other bits I forgot to get in Waitrose. I don't dawdle, for I'm eager to show my parents my new receptacle.

'What's that?' says Mum.

'It's for celery. It's a celery jar.'

'Oh. Well, it's going in a cupboard, it's hideous, Robert. It doesn't match anything in the kitchen.'

It doesn't match anything in existence, I think.

'Hang on,' says Dad, eyes widening, 'I think that was ours!'

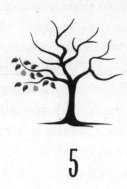

5

I like eating. I like it a lot. I'm a keen fan of chow. Big chewing enthusiast. What's this? A board of assorted cheeses in the middle of the night with a choice of chutneys? Yes, please, just let me fetch my cheese tools from my bedside drawer. I don't like the 'getting chubby' part of the deal, but thin doesn't feel nearly as good as fat tastes. At least, that's what I tell myself.

Therefore, it makes sense that I should attempt some kind of eating challenge. I've seen *Man v. Food*, all of them, repeatedly, and it looks like my kind of caper (mmm, capers). It's easy to find eating challenges in the US, Yanks are crackers for them. 'The Colonbuster Monster 5LB Texan Cowboy Challenge' pops up on American menus (on the Food Channel shows I watch, anyway) as regularly as fish and chips appears on British pub chalkboards. Most UK eating challenges seem to take place in greasy spoons and involve fry-ups the size of bin lids, heavily bulked out with triangles of patchily buttered white bread. You get a lot of variety with a cooked breakfast, so I suppose it makes sense to have them as challenge fodder – lots of tastes to keep you interested. A lot of moist to help sluice it down. But I fancy something a bit more Stars and Stripes. A towering burger, a giant pizza pie, a large dog (hot).

My flame-haired friend Adam, who I call B (surname: Bunker), and who calls me T, once attempted a burger-eating challenge with me at the Red Dog Saloon in London's Hoxton, a trendy place synonymous with creative types in vintage sports jumpers, putting stuff out in lower-case letters. Our mission: an eight-inch-tall, 3,000-calorie burger, to be consumed in ten minutes. I say we attempted it: in actual fact, we turned up and were told we hadn't booked, which was true, so we left. We scuffed our feet across the square to a bar. I left B at a table and went to the gents, returning to find him pressing himself flat against a wall, smashed glass covering the whole gaff. In the thirty seconds I'd been gone, two large gangs had sprinted into the place, gone behind the bar, had a bottle fight and then legged it out again. (That's what B told me had happened, anyway – perhaps he just had a rage attack.) It looked like the Ghostbusters had trashed the place trying to catch Slimer. But anyway, as far as food challenges go, I maintain that on that day, there was definitely an attempt. Of sorts.

I have eating-a-lot form. I nearly finished a 60 oz (1,700 g) steak on a work trip to Montreal, only stopping when I started hallucinating and had to go outside. I recently consumed eight large oranges in one sitting, resulting in tummy gripes so savage I considered going to A&E. In the end I was self-cured by an industrial amount of Rennie. Oh, and I tried to break the 'most bananas eaten in a minute' world record (six) in front of Guinness officials and my workmates at the time. Sadly I only managed half a banana. What else? I can eat three grab bags of Monster Munch and still have room for another regular-sized bag of Monster Munch. I'm not boasting, I just feel competitive eating might be my calling.

There's a retro diner down the A14, halfway to Cambridge. It's a sharp turn and rapid deceleration through a hand car wash to get there. There's nothing a 1950s-style diner enjoys more than hanging out by a busy A road. The diner, Herbies, is very *Happy Days*. Red booths, jukebox, probably a middle-aged man in a leather jacket who uses the toilet as his office. My nephew James likes the pancakes there. It offers a big burger challenge, and I will accept it. There's a massive Travelodge behind the restaurant in case I need to have a lie-down afterwards, or to simply burst in privacy.

Buddy Holly is playing in my car (I thought you were dead?!) to get me in an Americana mood, as I start the twenty-minute journey all giddy and raring to go, becoming increasingly tentative the closer I get until I'm sitting in the diner car park, watching lorries roar by, spraying dirty grey mist in their wake, wondering what the hell I'm doing with my afternoon. This is a silly plan. I have a sensitive pancreas (don't tell my pancreas I said that, it'll get upset) and fatty food won't do it any good. 'He Lost His Life Eating a Big Burger' isn't a legacy I fancy having. I watch the YouTube clip on my phone of someone from local radio attempting the challenge, and feel a bit repulsed. It's suddenly striking me as a revolting thing to do: quickly stuffing handfuls of soggy bread and mince into an already full mouth while saying 'oh god'. People in the world are starving. What a grotesque ambition. And it'll be well expensive. I know, somewhere inside me, probably my stomach, that too much food is bad, as is too little food. The best amount of food is a suitable amount. I think all of this in a dizzying loop and eventually decide not to do the challenge. Though I sort of know that I decided not to do the challenge when I was about halfway here, or possibly as soon as I set off. And I have a feeling I've reverse-engineered the whole safety/expense/morality excuse, and that the real reason I don't want to do it is because I don't want the attention. I'll feel embarrassed while attempting it, it'll be messy, I won't complete it anyway. It's pointless. It's not an adventure, it's a punishment. I've been in the car park for about an hour.

Eventually I just go for a drive. It's great to be able to drive again. I'd come to rely on a police-grade breathalyser I purchased online to check if I was safe to drive of a morning, and it usually said 'no', and there was no point even contemplating picking up my car keys come afternoon, so I solved the problem by simply staying in Godmanchester. In the car on my own is one of the few places I feel really at ease; razzing through the countryside, music turned up to just below the point when it starts to vibrate loose coins in the tray and slightly spoil each song. An Olly Murs–Snoop Dogg collaboration is sleazing its way out of the radio. It's one of those songs where men refer to women as 'señorita'. I'm not keen on the track, it's giving me bad vibes, so I go back to Spotify, still set on my US playlist. The soil of the ploughed fields I'm passing is so smooth they resemble giant lakes of hot chocolate. Johnny Cash sings about shiny shoes doing a million dollars' worth of good for you, which causes me to drive straight to the shops – I'm very suggestible – where I buy myself a pair of red leather brogues. A man of my age shouldn't be wearing tatty old Adidas trainers out and about. Because I'm not quite as reckless as someone like Johnny Cash, I also purchase some very strong leather protection spray. No rain damage for me. They look really sharp. Too nice to wear. I'll save them for a non-rainy day.

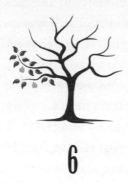

6

I'm on my way to Berlin for a few days with my friend Big Dan. I've decided to give solo travelling another go, but this time with another person.

Since the non-attempt at an eating challenge, I've had my head down for a few weeks, putting in a shift on the new *Very British Problems* book. My editor, Hannah, gave me some extra time, because of all that went on last year. These books are fun to do, and you don't need quite so thick a skin as you do with a popular Twitter feed, where random strangers, mostly young men, get in touch to tell you to die. Seriously. The last time this happened it was in response to a joke about the weather. Imagine becoming so cross over a Twitter account saying it's a bit rainy out. Very British Problems (or @SoVeryBritish) has rather typecast me a bit, as far as the opinions of the few people with enough time on their hands to be bothered about me personally go. Some people think I'm obsessed with tea (not that keen on it, actually, though I do drink a lot of it out of habit and politeness). Some think that I love the Queen (I am quite fond of those £20 notes she models for) and that I wear a bowler hat (head's too big for hats). Peculiar. I was even mistaken for the ombudsman of the English language at a Very British-themed book talk I was speaking at in Guildford. Getting myself to the event took a lot of courage, mostly the Dutch kind. I was terribly nervous on the train from Clapham Junction, the level of terror where you're almost in a trance. I stood in the wings as if about to take my turn at Live Aid, trying my usual trick of humming the 'nothing really matters, anyone can see' bit from 'Bohemian Rhapsody' to calm myself down. As usual, this trick didn't work; in a way, also as usual, it only heightened the wobbles. Floating on to the stage, I was sure I'd died and was having an out-of-body experience. I do not belong in front of an audience. To be honest, I can't remember much of this event, only the one strange question that came at the end of whatever I'd said for the last hour: 'I noticed you said "no worries" earlier. Do you think Australianisms and words from other countries are killing the English language?' Blimey. What a way to think. Words evolve and blossom from everywhere. New additions don't dilute language, only enrich it. What an answer that would have been! Instead I think I just said 'no'. Silence. Then I went to the lobby and sat in front of a pile of my books, while everyone filed past me and went home. But at least I'd done it, I suppose. Having never been on stage in my life, I'd just talked in front of a theatre full of strangers.

I have a love-hate relationship with Twitter. Without it, I might have a job I enjoy less, and I wouldn't be able to keep telling people, 'Hugh Laurie follows me, you know?' But it does suck you in. It can change you. I'm on Instagram, too, on a private account of just friends, but that's the real me. Wholesome, family me. Twitter me, on my personal account, is a character. A misanthrope. A grump. And I don't know who I'm playing this character for. It's distracting, unnecessary, attention-seeking madness, and I try to hold off indulging it as much as I can, but it's like trying to resist another wine gum when you've an open bag glued to your hand. Despite enjoying the process, I've still been putting off finishing the fourth *Very British Problems* book. It's a shame to start it in a way, because once you've started it'll soon be done, and when it's done, it's done. I'd like it to be in a state of permanent potential.

I did all my usual preflight preparations, and ordered a new portable battery charger, which turned out to be the size of a Bible. My iPhone only lasts about an hour these days, which is fine for when you sit permanently by a plug, which I have done for the past year or ten, but not when you're stomping around a city. I really should get a new phone. It's my main work tool, and it's held together by a rubber band. I popped into a phone shop in Huntingdon the other day with five minutes to spare before an appointment. A chap so young and fresh he made me feel mummified pounced and started nervously preaching all about the benefits of Three; I couldn't find a good place to cut him off and started to panic. I knew time was ticking away, like it does, because it was facing me on four different handsets. 'Okay ... okay, great, that's lovely, gotta dash but thanks for all your help (look at name badge) Ed!' Ed replied, 'Thanks, you too, Ed!' I could hear the sound of him dying inside.

I also ordered a new big coat. There is simply nothing better in life than a new big coat. You are for ever safe within a big coat. This coat is a navy (nearly all my clothes/possessions are navy) parka with fluffy hood. Seems to be the In Thing. I had it sent to Clifford's the Chemist.

'What's in the parcel?' The pharmacist and I are playing this game again.

'It's a jacket.'

'Yes, but what does it look like?'

'Kind of ... I don't know ... jackety?'

'Yes, but what shape is it?' The chemist makes big box/small box hand shapes.

'A box big enough for a jacket. It'll probably be folded. Look, I'm not being difficult, but I'm not really sure how to ...'

'What's the name again?'

'Temple.'

'Ah, here's one for a Temple. This must be it.'

While reaching into my wallet in Clifford's, an old fortune cookie fortune from Cinta fell out. *A fresh start will put you on your way.* I did what the fortune demanded and made myself go for a free trial at the Marriott Hotel gym a few miles down the A14. I hadn't seen Dan, or any of my friends, for a long time, so I told myself a single gym session would get me into 'looking good!' shape. I think it must be my face, or perhaps my paranoia, or both, but every time I approach any kind of reception desk and state the purpose of my visit, the person on the other side wears a bemused half-smile, as if I've rocked up in a jester hat and asked, 'Hello, is this where I come to buy the platypus?'

The gym is small, just one room, like most hotel gyms. It's off-white in colour and has a kind of medical vibe, like you'd come here for rehab. There's a row of step machines, a line of treadmills, a huddle of bikes, some free weights and four or five other machines. Also, a couple of balls, some mats, two rowing machines and two wall-size mirrors.

There are three older folks on machines and a couple of young, bulky chaps who appear to be there purely for the mirrors. They slowly pinball from one reflection to the other, as if trapped but feeling relaxed about it, much like goldfish. I use one of my three day passes to do an hour of lifting and pulling, then drive back to my parents' house to finish my packing. I find them discussing a new Martin Clunes drama. I always think of *Men Behaving Badly* when I think of Martin Clunes. It reminds me of my first-ever celeb interview with Neil Morrissey, who played Tony. For such a timorous person, I still question why I chose a career involving interviewing people. I had to wait until everyone had gone out for lunch before dialling the number. My voice was a trembling squeak. Neil Morrissey was remarkably kind to me and could tell I was nervous, probably because, instead of saying, 'I love you in *Men Behaving Badly*,' I accidentally just said, 'I love you.'

'I like Martin Clunes,' Mum said over her cup of tea. 'What else has he been in?'

'He was in *Men Behaving Badly*, Mum. You remember that?'

'No, no, I don't consider him Martin Clunes in that.'

The passport inspector in Berlin nods at me to step forward. How do they manage to look so cross? Why do they always seem so much more adult than me? 'Hello!' I chirp like a child. It's uncomfortable maintaining eye contact while they check that my face is definitely the older version of the face in the little maroon book I've just slid over. He stares at me and I can't help doing a little closed-mouth smile, basically raising everything on my face at once, the Brit-in-an-airport expression for 'I'm not a drug smuggler!' Dan's booked an Airbnb in Neukölln. It's late and dark (the two tend to go hand in hand) when we arrive. We have fish and chips for tea and call it a night.

In the morning it's still dark. And cold. And pissing it down. Undeterred, we head out for a day's trekking. A lot of Berlin seems to me like a big Shoreditch: if it was a level in the Crystal Maze it'd be called 'Industrial Hipster Metal Brick Cocktails Tiring Zone'. The rain's so relentless, it's making us wrinkle and steam. We decide to dry out over a couple of lunchtime bagels in one of the many small coffee shops. This one has church pews for seats. Soon we're having another big life chat. Dan talks while I listen, which is an arrangement we enjoy and have had since we met at university.

We shared our little first-year corridor in Nottingham (I tried to get into York but told the philosophy professor interviewing me, 'I feel it's important to feed the mind as well as the tummy.' You could crunch the silence like a toffee apple. Also, thanks to my careers adviser's insistence, I was wearing a suit, looking like I'd wandered in from filming *The Apprentice*) with Alex from Manchester, a lovely guy who gave away his bed to make more space in his room but then lacked a bed, and who used to cook a meal involving a can of tomato soup and chicken which he named 'Sexy Chicken'; Ian, a sporty chap (who had a dartboard on his side of the wall we shared) who in my memory always looks like Kevin Pietersen, and Chris M, a pleasant Britney Spears fanatic and perpetually paranoid engineering student, who convinced himself in our second year that our landlady was stealing our clothes through the wall via an invisible hole in the back of the washing machine. Gary and Dave, as well as Chris G, one of my closest mates from school, lived across the hall.

Dan got the nickname Big Dan to separate him from Little

Dan, who lived a floor up, and because he's big, resembling a polar bear. When he arrived on day one he unpacked bottles of every alcoholic spirit ever invented, from absinthe to vodka, as well as cocktail shakers and full barman paraphernalia, then introduced himself by telling me in a loud, posh, Oxford accent: 'If you touch any of my booze, I'll break your fucking legs.' He then complimented me on my sideburns. I was wary of him. He owned a cricket stump, named Lucille, which he'd routinely use to smash up the corridor wall, instructing visitors to do the same, proudly showcasing to all how soft the plaster was. I would then spend a lot of my time fixing the damage with filler so we'd retain our deposit in our self-catering accommodation, kept far away from the halls as if we were a virus. I had my doubts about whether we'd get on, but, like so many people you start off not really understanding, we've remained firm friends, and I have him to thank for getting me out of the house so many times during those three years. It's a role he's still committed to.

The first academic thing I had to attend on my English course was a 'meet and greet' – a truly horrible three words if ever there were. As we stood in a circle in the tutor's office, I heard those dreaded words echo around my head and instantly felt like being sick in my rucksack: 'Right, let's all go round, say a bit about our home towns and tell each other about our favourite book.' By the time it got to me, what seemed like four hours later, I managed to stutter, 'I won't say anything about my town because it's rubbish. And I like ... *Wuthering Heights.*' I very much do not like *Wuthering Heights*, it just popped into my head, like Ray from *Ghostbusters* thinking up the Stay Puft Marshmallow Man. I of course then started shaking like a jelly on a Power Plate. Everyone else looked cool and calm, like they'd been delivered straight from an episode of *Saved by the Bell*. The uni medical centre put me on beta blockers after that, and I put myself on red wine to help them dissolve.

Dan still refers to me as 7Up, a nickname I foolishly attempted to give myself in first year. When I'd fail to emerge from my pit for too many days, he'd walk me round the campus lake and make us pretend we were characters in *The Lord of the Rings*, commanding vast invisible armies stretching out to the horizon. We're cool guys. Getting out and about made me happier, who'd have thought? Seeing the daylight is nice sometimes, isn't it? But I can never do it without being dragged. Office life, and Rhi in particular, played a huge part in forcing and encouraging me to get a regular airing, but if I can get away with staying indoors then I will do just that. It wasn't until the past few years that I found out I could actually use 'anxiety' as a justification for it.

'You can't change who you are, 7Up, but you can change the things you do,' says Dan (which I'm sure is something Gandalf said) from the church pew he's squeezed into. 'But,' he continues, 'don't let those things that you do become your personality.' I'd just said I might get really into running again and run a hundred miles. He's right; running a long way won't magic me into an interesting person, it'll make me talk (a lot) about how I once ran a long way, which is the polar opposite of interesting. Yes, I know for a fact that that's exactly what happens ... my brother-in-law Pete and I did a couple of ultramarathons five or six years ago and I've never stopped mentioning it. See? 'How about if I cycle a hundred miles?' I ask, while staring out of the window. 'Are you only suggesting that because there's a bike chained to that lamp post that you're staring at through the window?' he replies.

'Maybe.' I can't decide whether it's wise to try to go back to extreme endeavours, or if I should be concentrating more on simply finding non-dangerous distractions that make me feel comfortable in my own skin. Is there such a thing as a healthy addiction?

Fuelled by bread, caffeine, Haribo and bars of Ritter Sport Joghurt, we march on through the concrete of Berlin in the downpour, an umbrella for Dan and a navy hood for me. I upload a few photos from our trip to Tempelhof Airport earlier in the day, while we have a Diet Coke in the café of the Gestapo HQ, which, unsurprisingly, sets the location of the photos as 'The Gestapo Headquarters'. Cripes. Delete! It's the last place you want people to think you've posed for a wacky 'A-HA!' Alan Partridge pose.

Dan subtly steers us around the city. He has a powerful undercurrent, possessing that skill of making a thoroughly planned day – oh, look, the Brandenburg Gate! – seem as if it's all just unfolding at random. It makes me feel safe, like I'm on a Scalextric track rather than freewheeling all over the road. Decisions are made for me as long as I keep saying 'I don't mind'. I like the automatic life; I like being a passenger if the driver is a pro. For the most part my phone stays in my pocket, coming out occasionally to take photographs, mostly of graffiti (won't look at those again) and check our step count. The sun sets as we pass the 50,000 mark. 'Why am I still fat?' I wonder. We stop into another coffee shop to dry off and warm up. It looks like it's been decorated by the Hyperion Antiques Centre. There's a juicer on a table with bird feathers sticking out of the funnel where you'd normally shove the fruit. Everyone in here is twenty-two and glaringly normcore. My breakfast tea arrives: a tall glass tumbler full of boiling water, balancing on a white saucer it doesn't even nearly fit, herbal teabag on the side and a sticky, nearly empty squeezy bottle of honey. If you want to really make it hit home to the customer that they've paid a few euros for a glass of hot water (which has to go cold before you can handle the glass), this is the way to do it. Dan has a coffee in a cup.

'So, now you're living the healthy life, you choose to go to one of the most debauched, decadent places in Europe?' laughs Dan. 'Where's next? Vegas?'

Vegas would be a fine choice with a good friend, I think, as we tidy the Airbnb, putting the complimentary water back in the lime-green fridge with the untouched complimentary cans of beer. If I went on my own I'd probably spend $10,000 on the minibar and room service burgers. If Dan and I went, we'd march up and down the strip, occasionally stopping for tea and biscuits. On the flight home, we're all talked out, and communicate only by tilting our phones at each other to show what songs we're listening to on Spotify.

'Well, you know where I am, buddy,' Dan says at the airport. 'Stay in touch.' And with that he's off, putting his headphones in and giving his customary backwards wave – as if about to high-five an invisible person in front of him – as he walks away. It's been a fine adventure.

Back in Godmanchester, I discover that Dad's bought a big pile of soil, as tall as a car. 'It's £270! If you buy it from a company it costs six hundred quid. I got this from a client for £270.' We stare at the soil, newly dumped in his driveway. I can't fathom spending literally hundreds of pounds on mud. 'Have you ever seen soil that orange before?' asks Mum. I've never. We all stand and stare at the soil for a bit longer, then Dad gets a call from the hospital about Mum's medication, the securing of which has been a palaver. I cover the soil with tarp and weigh it down with bricks. Later, Dad sets about it with the shovel. Shovelling soil looks quite fun – not that I join in. Shovelling, chopping, chainsawing and possibly lawn-mowering are all 'God Tier' gardening. As long as there's not too much bending, I'm all for it. As yoga proved, I'm naturally quite rigid and also idle, so no gardening at all is preferable. 'You must remember to go to the toilet before you use the wheelbarrow,' I hear Mum say to Dad as I walk towards the house. 'It's harder to lift with a full bladder.' Later, Dad comes in for tea.

It's freezing out there. Spring still seems a long way off. The crumble's all gone for another year, so we've reverted back to the usual pudding: yoghurts. Disappointing compared to crumble.

'What yoghurt do you want, Mum?'

'What is there?'

'Cherry, strawberry, toffee, vanilla, cranberry and raspberry together.'

'Say them again?'

'Cherry, strawberry, toffee, vanilla, cranberry and raspberry together.'

'I'll have cherry.'

'Okay. Dad?'

'What?'

'What yoghurt do you want?'

'What is there?'

'Cherry, strawberry, toffee, vanilla, cranberry and raspberry together.'

'I don't mind.'

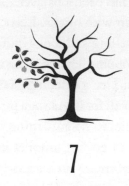

7

I'm trapped in the jelly in a big pork pie. It's comfortable and warm, being suspended in the squishy window betwixt meat and pastry. I hope nobody cuts through me with a huge shiny knife. No, they wouldn't do that. I'm safe in my pie. I'm in a womb. I'm being harvested for energy. I've seen *The Matrix*, I know what they're up to. But I don't mind, I don't mind at all. I'm in a butcher's womb. What? A sexy butcher. Weird. It's nice. Oh. Okay. Because I'm a warm egg. Help. Imagine if there was a dog in here with me ... on a special li-lo. Imagine if the water was Worcestershire sauce. Hope it's Lea & Perrins. There's a sea bass in here with me. I'm the first pork pie in space, heading to Mars.

When I heard that your mind plays surreal tricks in a flotation tank, I expected my own to come up with something a little more profound than 'I'm in a pie'.

Before I came to this tank to lie down in water, I was doing a drier version in a bed, waking – in the oversized, tatty, holey, WAKE UP AND LIVE-emblazoned bed T-shirt I've had since I was fifteen – at the crack of 7.25 a.m. to drive to meet Lisa, my older sister, by a barn on a farm in Ware. I'm determined to achieve a state of zen. Surely that's the goal of doing most things, to reach contentment, to be happy in your own skin if only for an hour, or a few minutes? I tend to find my skin about as comfortable as sitting on German church pews. I carry myself like four plastic pint glasses. Yoga might zenify me if I stick at it, but I need the quick, legal hit of relaxation only being a vegetable in a big pan of salty broth can promise.

Lisa and Pete live halfway between me and London, with my nephew, Finlay, and niece, Freya, both teens. Lisa's the ideal partner for a flotation challenge – she's big into well-being. She doesn't drink, eats a keto diet and exudes health and positivity; much less of a mis hog than me. 'I can't help but think I'm commuting for an hour in order to take a warm bath,' I'd said to Dad this morning by the kitchen door, as he stood at the sink downing a tall glass of tap water. He very much treats the need for liquid as if he's a car, filling himself up from the nozzle and then going until empty, rather than the modern fashion of being constantly topped up with bottled Volvic. 'Well, that's the power of marketing for you, paying to have a bath,' he replied, ushering me out through the back door into the cool spring air. To be fair to Float UK, they haven't marketed this adventure to me at all – I went looking for them online. Floating in a small pool of Epsom salts is, I've read, very close to being in zero G, and, therefore, nice. All your muscles relax, even more so than in bed, because nothing needs support. Even sitting on your arse all day requires some effort from your arse. Flotation takes that burden away.

Speaking of bed, although I paid north of £50 for my sister

and me to bob around for half an hour (in separate tanks), it'd been the usual battle to convince my lazy brain that leaving my mattress was worth it (how lazy is that? Too lazy to stop lying down to go somewhere else to lie down). At that perfect level of early-morning warmth after a peaceful night's sleep, you feel at one with Duvet. And yes, the proper name usage was intentional. You're the banana and it is the peel. But stay in bed all morning and people become concerned, whereas travel through rush hour traffic down the A1 for sixty minutes to pay by debit card to recline in some warm H_2O and people say, 'Wow, tell me more, you sound like a pure pleasure seeker.' Of course, the best thing about having a lie-in is that you wake up with less time to wait until lunch. Carpe diem, my arse. Carpe pillow.

I love sleeping. I had so many years when I couldn't. Torture! Bed is no place to be awake by yourself. I still have sleepless nights now and then, kept awake by a whirring mind, but nowhere near the wide-eyed, leg-twitching madness of the last two years. I also near nightly have that classic anxiety dream of being about to take exams that I haven't revised for. In my case it's A-levels, and throughout the dream I'm arguing with the teachers that I'm in my thirties and shouldn't still be in school ... 'This is madness! I've already passed these!'

I especially love sleeping in moving vehicles. I never resist the feeling of unconsciousness coming to take me. When sleep is coming, the heavy kind that feels like it should be accompanied by an anaesthetist's countdown, I let my eyes fall like car bonnets and go with it, wherever I am. Nothing comfier than a nap. Bus sleeping is best, wrapped in a big coat at 10 a.m., hands wrapped around a hot paper coffee cup, windows misted with condensation, the faint scent of diesel coming and going. The wheels go round and round as your thoughts disperse like the final effervescent bursts of a Berocca, and then nothing, nothing but the engine's gentle vibration, rocking you into oblivion. Wonderfully drugged. The only downside is waking up somewhere new with a stiff neck like a fat man's been sitting on it. Anyway, I'm hoping flotation might be a bit like that.

After Google Maps – which Mum once described as a 'silly sod' for giving her duff directions – deposits me in various bright yellow fields, I turn into the correct field and park. The aroma of grass floats in the air, so strong it could be emanating from a high-end scented candle. I stare at some cows and they stare back. Lisa arrives five minutes later, albeit still pleasingly early.

'Hello, how are you?'

'Hellooo!' beams Lisa.

Hug.

'I've got some Easter eggs in the car from Mark, he says sorry they're late.' I bundle two Thorntons boxes that've been thrown around my back seat on the twisty drive here into Lisa's arms; she puts them in her Skoda Yeti. I can't believe it's May already. March and April were spent recuperating after another spell in Bay Tree Ward. I'd thrown myself off the wagon with quite some force, aggravating my pancreas in the process. Rhi came to the hospital to visit me, and we had a long chat about the divorce. Later I realised I'd hallucinated the whole meeting, a not-so-fun effect of severe alcohol withdrawal. I also became convinced that a featureless man sitting at the end of my bed, called Jimmy Smiles, was trying to convince me to help him run a Motown record label, while a hectic drum solo played from nowhere.

'Sorry I'm late, I forgot my swimming costume. I kept worrying I was going the wrong way,' says Lisa.

'Same, it really is in the middle of nowhere, isn't it?'

We stand in front of the barn. If not for the big Float UK sign and the fact that the barn has a doorbell, we'd look remarkably, comically lost. We wait until 9.45 a.m., fifteen minutes, as suggested, before our appointment, and ring the bell. A young woman in sports kit opens the door and welcomes us into the dimly lit, windowless, peaceful, spa-like reception. Once inside it's hard to fathom that outside is all hay and farm as the scent switches from grass and cow to herbal tea and fresh towels. It all smells a bit swimming pool.

'Are you first-time floaters?' We've never been asked before. 'Yes,' we reply, though I want to ask, 'Do we *look* like first-time floaters?!'

'Great, if you'd like to come through here and fill out the forms, then I'll take you upstairs and show you how it all works.'

In the 'Relaxation Lounge' we give our details and agree to the rules, which include no smoking in the tanks and no contaminating the water with organic waste 'thus causing an incident'. Once contractually obliged not to poo ourselves (if the person who made this written rule necessary is reading, shame on you), we trot upstairs. The advice goes roughly thus: have a shower, get dry, once the tank (about the size of a very small hatchback) fills up with water, get in, shut the door, lie there until the light and music come back, try not to get salt in your eyes, shower again, done. We're silently stumped by some overly complicated tank door shutting and opening instructions and I can tell Lisa isn't taking it in, and neither am I, because I'm watching Lisa not taking it in, so we begin our floats fearing we'll be trapped in our respective tanks indefinitely. After thirty minutes – though it seems like five – we manage to exit our pies, sorry, tanks and meet up again in the Relaxation Lounge for herbal teas.

'How did you get on?' I ask.

'Yeah, I loved it.'

'Same, really good.'

'Although at first I was in there widthways.'

'Widthways?'

I can't really work out how this is possible without being folded tightly in half, so I'm glad to hear Lisa soon changed to lengthways for the sake of her vital organs.

And it *was* nice, such as it was. It felt relaxing not to be worrying about the past or the future. Nice not to be worrying about time passing. Time flies whether or not you're having fun; shame to dwell on it. When I get a bit morose about . . . stuff, my solution, albeit a rather crude and sometimes ineffective one, has always been to drown those thoughts, to ignore them, to hide them away somewhere in my mind, back where they came from. Fingers in ears, lalala I can't hear you. Flip the thoughts over like wine stains on cushions. The stains are still there, of course, there's no doubting them, but they don't always have to spoil the room. I sweep so many things under the rug that it's nearly touching the ceiling. I know repression in general isn't all that healthy (or is it?) but sometimes you have to just crush your thoughts before they crush you.

As well as flotation being like a peaceful nap, I also anticipated it to be a bit like a counselling session (if you're reading this, Ruth, I'm sorry – I just equated speaking to you with lying in a shallow patch of salty water). I expected to 'work through' a few troubling thoughts, put them into order and gain some perspective, but my experience was wholly akin to the meandering dreams you get before drifting off. Physically it felt pleasant, too, even if I was a bit embarrassed to be naked in front of myself. I'd glance down at my body in the tank to see I resemble Chas, Morph's pale friend, dead in a canal. Should've worn trunks. It's not really a hobby, though, floating, unfortunately. Not like metal-detecting or getting really into coffee or polishing surfaces. I can't do it at home. I mean, I suppose I could make my own tank out of an old chest freezer, but that's got 'funeral' written all over it. I'll never be a first-time floater again, but outside of a flotation tank facility I can't imagine I'll ever proudly describe myself as 'a floater'. Others might.

Driving home through the bright fenland countryside, I'm thinking of the marketing work for Pimm's I have to finish off. I'd love a bottle of Pimm's. Stepping through the door, I receive a WhatsApp from Lisa: the words 'probably the most boring photo I've ever taken in my life' on a picture of eight large white sacks of salt at the bottom of a staircase. I quite like it.

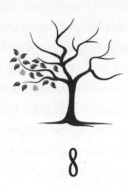

8

'*Elle come manzanas*,' I mutter into my phone, while searching the fresh produce aisles of Tesco for berries, seeds and bracken. '*Bebo leche*,' I softly growl, as I meet the terrified eyes of a young mother choosing broccoli. It's unfortunate that the strict owl who rules over the language-learning app Duolingo, has decided that *NOW NOW NOW!!!* is the best time for my Spanish lesson. I fear I'm about to be accosted by security for accusing women of stealing apples.

I've always wanted to learn another language. Well, always wanted to *speak* another language, I'm not thrilled about the learning part. I 'did' GCSE French at school, so I tell people I know enough French to get by, which is simply a lie. Unless by 'get by' I mean pointing at a swimming pool and naming it. It's the same deal as if you went to the sort of school, as I did, that insists rugby is an essential life skill; you tell people, 'I used to be a prop,' well into old age, even though you were only eight at the time and about as much use on a sports field as a dead lamb. I still tell rugby tales, such as when Mr Barton threw a pupil a clear ten metres over the rugby posts, allegedly the standard punishment for not being good in a ruck, even though it never actually happened. It's hard to remember what's myth and what's reality with Mr Barton. Spending most of your early schooldays being tackled into freezing mud messes up your memory. I do remember he would begin every house meeting, in classrooms that memory will have me believe were made completely of expensive wood, by throwing undergarments, abandoned or lost in the changing rooms, at whoever matched the sewed-in name tag inside. It was like the scene in *Full Metal Jacket* where the drill sergeant is assigning everyone their jobs, but with boxer shorts instead of roles. 'Smith ... infantry. Stevens ... infantry. Temple ... pants.' Then I'd have to retrieve my flung Y-fronts from the nearby head they'd landed on. I also remember a teacher pushing us back into the showers with a broom if we weren't clean enough after practice.

If we weren't busy playing rugby or losing/regaining pants, we were busy, from the age of about nine, writing with fountain pens, wearing beige trench coats over our little suits and carrying briefcases. They were creating weird mini businessmen. It's a wonder we didn't have business cards: 'Rob Temple, Small Boy'. So yes, anyway, the upshot of my education is that I'm a retired professional rugby player and fluent in French. I fancy being fluent in Spanish now. Oh, and I'm also vegan as of this morning. Both these adventures require only self-discipline, training and work ethic – there's no audience, there's no exam ... so they should be easy-peasy.

Yesterday, while I was eating scrambled chicken zygote on toast, I looked up at the Sunday papers to see the headline: 'Shall I join the stampede to turn VEGAN?' Dr Michael

Mosley, pictured wielding a Greggs vegan sausage roll – a snack recently made famous by virtue of Piers Morgan being furious at it – claimed that 500,000 people in Britain were now plant-based. Half a million, all based in plants. 'Why aren't I plant-based?' I thought. Sounds like an adventure to me. Mosley, make that 500,001 (please).

Sunday p.m. turned to Monday a.m. as I stood in pyjamas in the chilly glow of the fridge stuffing my chops with mature cheddar and fistfuls of leftover roast chicken, before going to bed for my last meat-sweating, nightmarish cheese sleep. For a fortnight, anyway. I'm only doing a two-week tester run, see. I'm wearing my V-plates (meant something different at school). Cards on the table, I really like eating meaty, non-vegan (Megan?) stuff. I don't need to eat animal products, I have the time and the resources to avoid them and still enjoy a salubrious diet. I eat animals because I have a long list of favourite foods involving milk and limbs, and I'm selfish, so there you go. Unfortunately you can't decide you're powerless over chomping flesh; you have to own the greediness. If I lose a bit of weight by cutting down on my frankly astonishing mayo intake, I might continue with veggie life. I'm teetering like a bus on the cliff edge of sixteen stone. My silhouette in profile seems to be that of a melted candle. As A. A. Milne wrote, 'A bear, however hard he tries, grows tubby without exercise'. And I've a wedding to attend in a few months, ergo I have a suit to get into (I can't afford to keep buying a new one for every wedding), so my vanity could save at least a whole cow. Plus I can start chatting about veganism at the reception if I'm tired and want to be left alone.

'So are we all going vegan, then?' Dad asks sadly after I break the news of my plan.

'You don't have to, Dad, but I'm going to try it.'

'Don't worry about him, he'll eat what he's given,' says Mum. 'And if you don't like it, Paul, you can always add non-vegan things to your meals.'

'Am I allowed ham?'

'If you want ham you can have ham. I've seen M&S do a big vegan range now. Ooh, we'll have to get some almond milk to have in tea.'

Dad looks like he's been deeply insulted.

'Well, I'm having normal milk in my tea, thank you very much, I don't care what you say.' Dad has almond milk for the next fortnight.

I don't expect my folks to change their diets, but Mum insists – she likes joining in, and she hopes a fruitier intake might help with her arthritis, and Dad can't cook, so he's just a bit stuck with it. I also state that I, intrepid mild adventurer that I am, won't be doing any fancy-pants ready meal veganism: I'll be living on that which grows upon tree and shrub. I'm a forager, nature is my pantry. Plus, I've had bad experiences with pretend meat the last six or seven times I've gone veggie. For years I had a freezer full of fake sausages and burgers. I couldn't find a range I was particularly keen on. Even tried to palm them off on Raffy. He stared at the fake sausage on the floor and then looked sadly at me, as if to say, 'I'm not angry with you, I'm just disappointed'. I'm talking about a dog who would go out of his way to try and eat wood and poo no matter how much I tried to convince him it wasn't part of a balanced diet.

'And where will you be getting all this nature from?' asks Mum, while coating the entire kitchen in Lavender Escape-scented Zoflora.

'Tesco.'

I find it quite hard to imagine a week's worth of meals when I'm just staring at rows of vegetables. I think simplistically in meat-and-two-veg plate design, which is now veg-and-two-veg. I'll have to go to my backup cooking method: one pot. *'Ella es un bebe,'* I whisper at the mushrooms. More worried looks. *'Bebo ... agua.'*

A supermarket conveyor belt heaving with colourful veg looks good. Smugness sloshes over me like a full bath of tepid oat milk. So this is why vegans do it. (Joking: I know it's not why you do it, oh FOR THE LOVE OF GOD you've already written in, haven't you? And I know the whole humourless thing is a stereotype, but stereotypes come from somewhere. I could just delete the joke, but then that'd be me thinking you'd be sensitive about it, which would be pushing the stereotype even more, wouldn't it? Or maybe you are humourless, in which case, fair enough, having a sense of humour isn't mandatory. You may be a vegan with a sense of humour who simply didn't find the joke amusing, also fair enough. I mean, statistically speaking, you're reading this, thinking 'I'm not even a vegan', so I'm making a fuss about nothing. How have we got here? I've had four coffees, that's how. I'm sorry.)

'Still raining out there?'

'Yes, awful, isn't it?'

'I don't mind it.'

'No, me neither, I love it.'

'I wouldn't go that far. Do you need any help packing?'

'Erm ...' I know I'm going to say no. 'No, I think I'll be okay, thank you.'

'Do you need any bags?'

I look at all my bags. 'I miiight do . . . I'll see how I get on.' Friendly chuckle.

'Yeah, meant to be raining all weekend, they say.'

'Typical, isn't it?'

'Well, no, it's been lovely up till now.'

I get home with such goods as a bag of sweet potatoes (sweet potato will become a close friend in the next few weeks), a bunch of bananas, a small packet of tofu, mushrooms, a rainbow of peppers, a squat plastic tub of tomato and basil pasta sauce, balls of pickled beetroot, some vegan vanilla ice cream and cartons of various not-milks. I think I need some recipes. Of course I make a formal announcement on Instagram about my new lifestyle – what's the point in being quietly vegan? And while we're on the subject, has anyone ever bought a veg box without telling anyone? How would we know? I'm over the moon by how delighted some of my plant-munching friends are at the news. Natasha congratulates me, Tori gives me a 'YAS!!!' and my cousin Nicola invites me to her separate and secret vegan Instagram profile full of recipes. I feel like a newcomer being welcomed to church. Either all the chlorophyll has sent my friends doolally, or there's something in this. I have a feeling a new me awaits.

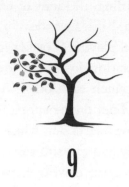

9

'They're all over the country. You just register online and then you show up and run. It's free, I have a lot of clients who do it.' Lauren's telling me about Parkrun while I tremble my way through another thirty-second plank. 'Sounds a bit like AA but for running,' I reply. 'You get a free T-shirt when you've done something like fifty runs,' she adds. Sold. Sounds like a pleasant adventure, and I love a free T-shirt.

I'm back on it with the personal training. It's expensive, more so than a gym membership, anyhow, but then not nearly as much as I used to spend in the off-licence. Since I last saw her – must be getting on for a year ago now – Lauren, my personal trainer, has moved her training sessions from Godmanchester to Bills Gym at the very end of a business park in St Neots, surrounded by Realfit, Peppercorns Music Academy and New Saints Amateur Boxing Club. Bills is a real boxing gym! People box there and everything. It has a boxing ring. It's like the gym in *DodgeBall*. On the bright and sunny twenty-minute drive here this morning, my mind is going haywire, swirling all kinds of nonsense around. 'I wonder if Bill will be at Bills. I wonder if it'll be Bill Clinton.' I imagine Bill Clinton playing 'Love Is In The Air' (but in my head I'm singing 'spring' instead of 'love') on a sax in the corner while people punch each other. A strange thought, and one I don't enjoy. I put on my upbeat 'Drive' playlist and 'Walking On Sunshine' blasts out, which I find ludicrously over the top, especially in a car, so I turn it off. It's so maniacally happy, I can imagine driving casually off a cliff to it with a big grin on my face.

Upon arrival, I'd like to say I accidentally went into the wrong door, that I entered Peppercorns Music Academy and started bench-pressing a double bass in front of horrified children. But this wouldn't be true. I walked through the correct door – exactly on time, after loitering round the corner and counting down the seconds on my watch – then along a corridor that smelled of lemon bleach and into a land of punchbags. I've never seen a boxing ring in the flesh before, but here it is, looking just like a boxing ring. Pictures of Tyson and Ali and other boxers plaster the walls. The floor is pink and spongy and what I only know as 'Ibiza music' pumps from a stereo. It's empty apart from one person doing a workout (not Rocky, unfortunately). I gently thump a punchbag and watch as it doesn't move a millimetre, as if I've just thumped a wall. I haven't even taken my fleece off yet, and already I've probably broken my wrist in three places. The immediate temptation to feel the ropes of the boxing ring is almost too much to bear, but I worry I might set off some kind of alarm, or that the man doing his workout might see it as a signal to fight him.

Lauren has me deadlifting, rowing, lunging, doing

embarrassing thrusting ('Really fire those hips through!'), stretching, grunting my way through an hour of gentle exercises that see me lying and panting on the deck (you can really see every hair and speck of dirt on the floor when your face is pressed against it), at times sure that I'm dead. If you want to feel really uncomfortable, if you're me, then try thrusting your hips while you lie on your back with your feet atop a big inflatable ball; I haven't been that embarrassed since I was packed off to school with a brand-new tan leather rucksack and my games kit in a Harrods bag. In this gym I use some of my muscles for the first time, like, ever, so I spend a lot of the 'just get your breath back' time vibrating like a fish freshly chucked on land.

Lauren's been a student at some of the country's top ballet schools and has performed on telly and all sorts. She can nonchalantly bend in ways that would permanently hamper my ability to walk if I tried them. Despite her size (S), I've no doubt she could body-slam all 200 lbs-plus of me into the canvas, should I anger her with my poor planking form. Her website states: 'Because of my dancing background, my training approach focuses a lot around core and postural work, as well as correction of form and technique for full body balance'. That's good for me, as I have none of these. In fact, I think my core is about as firm as a trifle, and would probably explain the main cause of all my past running injuries as a younger, lighter man. 'Anyway, see what you think of Parkrun. I know a lot of people who love it.'

I'm in Hinchingbrooke park with all the people. So many people; 254 people, to be exact, all milling about, stretching, looking cold, waiting for 9 a.m. to roll around. I'm among them, waiting to start my first Parkrun. If I can't get my zen through flotation, then maybe I'll have to work harder for it. I've had the runner's high before, but as I mentioned in Berlin, I took it too far to maintain (woe are my poor knees!) with the ultramarathons. Three miles is perhaps more my distance. I'll be a mild-mannered reporter in the weekdays, go to bed at a normal hour, wake at a normal hour, then at the weekend bosh out three miles in a park with other runners, then have a roast dinner and walk a dog. Sounds normal. Maybe normal is good. I should stop trying to make an easy life hard with extremes. I'm not an extremes guy. An anxious mind, I suppose more than anything in my case, seems to simply present life as much more complicated than it actually is or indeed has to be. I halt plans to dig out all my specialist running kit and buy an antigravity treadmill and make room for my future ironman tattoo. In fact, somewhere I've got a metal medal holder that says 'Always Forward Progress' or something, from my marathon days (runners seem to need constant reminders that forward is the necessary direction of travel). I never attached it to the wall, though. Couldn't be bothered.

'You're making a right meal of those socks,' Mum says, as I sit on the sofa and struggle to wrench them on. The last time I attempted to apply these fancy, too-expensive socks, years ago, my grip slipped and I punched myself in the balls. Now I hold onto them for dear life. I struggle with socks at the best of times, but seeing as compression socks would fit tightly on a pencil, getting them on my legs is an unattractive ordeal.

'Is anyone here doing their first run?' a lady says through a microphone connected to a loudspeaker that's not working. A few people put their hands up while my hand stays down, the liar. 'Make your way over there.' Off I go to join the splinter group of newbies. We're told the Parkrun rules, which, to paraphrase, are:

1. Run or walk the 5K at your leisure.
2. If you haven't got your printed barcode (mine's stuffed inside my glove – hopefully I won't sweat away all the ink) or fancy wristband (yesterday they'd released a purple one, a colour I'd read online had been named the Pantone Colour of the Year. I should get this one, I think), then you won't get a time at the end.
3. I miss this rule, as I'm too busy thinking about the colour purple.
4. If you're under eleven, you have to be with an adult. A responsible one. I look at my watch to note that, sadly, I've been over eleven for twenty-two years.
5. Don't push any dog walkers into the lake, etc.

We're told the course route, but, reassured that unless we plan to run the distance in seventeen minutes or less, we're best off just following the person in front. I suspect I won't be leading the pack unless I do it on a motorbike (Rule 6, which I'm pretty sure is unwritten, is no motorbikes).

I'm reasonably confident as I wait at the Parkrun starting line that I'll be able to cover the 5K distance without keeling over. I might be pushed over, though, as I've made the rookie mistake of standing at the front. This is where the speedsters start, I learn, as they all stream past me at 90 mph. But soon I'm running with my people, the determined plodders. Here I am, after years of nothing, keeping pace with a group of strangers again. As we stomp around the pretty, lakeside, two-lap course, I feel … I don't know, some sort of peace, maybe? I'm newly wary of getting too optimistic, so I just tell myself that I feel 'not bad'. After a night of small panics – would I get here on time? Will I do something wrong? Is it really for me? What if I mess everything up? It's literally moving from A to B: imagine if you mess that up! – I'm jogging down a path thinking of breathing and moving, and that's about it. At this moment, I'm just caught up in running, surrounded by people. And I'm okay. Other runners say, 'You're doing well, mate' as they pass; volunteers clap as they shout, 'Good running, keep going!' It feels good to be told to keep going, and I try to pay it forward. 'Keep it up,' I offer to precisely one person (hearing my own voice say 'keep it up' actually annoys me a bit, if I'm honest, but at least I say it), and I make sure I thank the volunteers as I pass. As I say, it's chat set to 'Beginner'.

I'd tweeted that I'd be at the Parkrun a few days earlier as a way of making sure I had every urge to make it to that starting line. I find this strategy often helps. 'Motivation through fear of awkwardness since 1983', I said in the tweet. I'd copied in @parkrunUK and they, or more accurately 'someone', kindly replied, 'It's a date, Rob. And looking at the weather (obviously), you can leave that British brolly at home, too'. This is how people speak to me now, by the way, like I'm a brand. I don't mind, it's to be expected; I just find it quite funny. I do the same to others on social media. I tweeted my love of Robinsons Apple & Blackcurrant squash to Robinsons as if the person in charge of tweeting back also really loves squash. They might hate squash, for all I know; it's just a job (I was sent a free bottle of squash in the post, though, so it was worth it).

I'm keeping an eye on my left knee. It's a dodgy one. Lauren highly suspects this is because my calves are hyperextended. You find this out by standing straight with your legs locked. If they go straight down to the ground below the knee, you have regular old legs. If they bow out backwards, they're hyperextended. 'Would you mind standing up and showing me your legs?' I'd said to a friend on meeting for coffee the other day. 'Yeah, you see, your legs are normal,' I replied, with a hint of disappointment in my voice. We sat down and waited for our drinks, her not quite sure what had just happened.

Anyway, what I now term 'hyper legs' basically means I'm putting a lot of pressure on the front part of my knee, which could lead to pain. I've been advised to try to stand with my legs slightly bent whenever possible. Have you tried standing with your legs a bit bent? It looks bizarre. A bit creepy. But anyway, I'd tried to remember the advice leading up to this run, crouching down whenever I was doing something like chopping veg, cleaning my teeth, having a wee, and I'm pleased to note that I'm not feeling any pain on the Parkrun. Turns out bendy legs like mine are quite sought after in ballet, by the way, so maybe I'll just pirouette the whole way.

I'm also keeping the feelers (what are feelers?) out for any pain in my Achilles tendons, the huge strings round the backs of the ankles, which in the past have made alarming twanging sounds. Apparently you send the force of about seven times your body weight through these when you're pounding the ground, which in my case would be the weight of half a car. Lauren said we'd do some metatarsal strengthening exercises – such as calf raises – to try to give the Achilles a bit of help. And hopefully oats will provide enough power to take me the distance. I'd usually have a piece of toast for breakfast. Sometimes with an egg on it. Sometimes with bacon on it, too, and sometimes with another piece of toast on top. This morning, once my socks were finally on, I had porridge. I hate porridge. Some people love it. They literally say, 'Mmm, I love porridge.' To me it seems like saying 'I love shoelaces', or 'I love pointing at things'. It's just something that 'is'. Not to be enjoyed. Maybe I'm making it wrong. Mum sometimes sprinkles flaxseed on hers, from a large sachet in the cupboard. It looks like a rollie-smoking student has turned his trouser pocket inside out over the bowl. Nice and gritty. Porridge is also very tricky to eat in a hurry when you're worried you're late. You can't clench a half-eaten bowl of wet oats in your mouth as you grab your bag and keys and rush to the car, like they do in the adverts with toast. You'd look untrustworthy.

Quick look at my app ... a third of the way round. Feeling okay. Legs very muddy, but I'm sure it'll come off. 'Keep going, mate!' 'Ta!' 'Well done!' 'Morning!' 'Not far now, pal!'

I'm daydreaming about windscreen wipers. I wonder if people who design cars wish there was a more technical solution to wiping water off a big piece of glass. Do they get annoyed that it's 2019, and we're still relying on two brushes on big sticks literally scraping away the wet at speeds ranging from slow to 'we're gonna die!'? I reckon if there was some kind of ... hang on, is that the finish line? It bloody is. Out of nowhere, only about fifty yards in front of me! People are cheering, various neon jerseys are shooting by trying to crack their personal bests, the sun is shining. My mind has reached that blissful state of becoming so relaxed that it actually wanders to idle thoughts, rather than the irrational worries it harbours for most of the day. Cheaper than being a floater! More effort, mind. During the course of the run I'd moved from panic, to thinking about my breathing, to breathing automatically while in a kind of trance and pondering nothing of any importance whatsoever. To have a brain ticking over rather than darting around like it's on *Supermarket Sweep* is nice.

I look at my app to discover I've got a personal best: my fastest 5K of the year! It's my only 5K of the year, but still, sounds pretty professional. A text comes through. 'Rob, your time in position 164 today at Huntingdon Parkrun was 32:19. Well done on your first run here'. It dawns on me that I've done something good today. I feel like smiling. Smiling on the inside, obviously; I don't smile when I'm on my own, I'm not that strange. I feel good, though. Kind of light. Is the runner's high back? I wouldn't go that far. Perhaps more a kind of relief. Maybe I could just keep running for ever, like Forrest Gump.

Now, how do I make the feeling I get during and immediately after running stick around? I'm sure it used to be more powerful, longer-lasting, when I was younger. Perhaps because I did more of it. I can't just run for ever. Or maybe I could? Forrest did it. But then again, he was a character. Mustn't get carried away.

'How hard do you reckon it is to run 100 miles?' I text Lauren. 'Do you think it's double?'

'Yes, as long as you build up slowly. You won't run 100 miles until the actual day, either.'

'Ah, right,' I say, casually, as if being told the dishwasher needs emptying.

'The most important thing for you will be stretching.'

'And running?'

'Yes, running and stretching. I can make you strong, but you have to stretch. And run.'

'It's a long way though, isn't it, 100 miles?'

'A very long way,' she confirms. She doesn't seem too worried. I imagine she's heard plans like this from many a 35-plus man, who then disappears after two sessions. Or, more likely, she just knows what she's doing.

A text comes through from Mark, on his lunch break.

'So have you really joined a boxing gym in St Neots?'

News travels fast round these parts.

'Yeah.'

'Lol, finding that hard to picture.'

'What's hard to picture? I'm like a young Sly Stallone. I might buy a grey tracksuit and start drinking eggs at 4 a.m.'

'Yeah, you do that.'

Wait . . . is it safe to drink eggs?

'Is it safe to drink eggs?'

'It's not advisable. Tastes bad. Besides, they only take a minute to cook.'

'I will drink the eggs. Oh ye of little faith' (something I like to say, particularly before I let someone down).

'Go for it.'

'Actually, I'm not allowed eggs.'

Maybe I could run 100 miles. Maybe I should try boxing. Maybe . . . something else. I spend the best part of the rest of the morning thinking and trying to chisel bits of dried oats from a cereal bowl. Perhaps I should just try to commit to doing at least two Parkruns a month. Yes, it's worth a try.

10

I've finished being vegan. For the first few days I was bursting with all the expert knowledge of the newcomer – after two or three days of blindly but enthusiastically stumbling your way through anything, you know it all: everything's meatless gravy in the pink cloud phase. Then, well, I'll be honest, I just really wanted a burger after doing such a long run through the park, and I couldn't put up enough resistance. There's nothing more to it than that, sadly. I'm not proud of it, I just have an extreme lack of willpower. I'll definitely try to reduce my animal intake from now on, though. I shouldn't be eating meat every day, it's just a ridiculous thing to do. I'll give vegetarianism a proper go at some point, I'm sure of that. I like to think I've learned a few things the past fortnight, most of them probably quite obvious to most people.

Vegan pros:

- Choice: there's loads of choice! Supermarkets even have their own burgeoning plant-based sections, and that's as well as the acre of fruits and veggies! In Costa I absent-mindedly ordered a latte. Just as the chap was heading to the fridge, I, a rank vegan amateur, blurted out, 'Oh, sorry sorry sorry I forgot, I'm meant to be vegan.' He didn't miss a beat (there must be another vegan in Huntingdon) when replying, 'We've got almond milk, soy, coconut ... actually I think we're out of coconut, and lactose-free.' How cool is that? I mean, you probably already know about all this, but it was a revelation to me. I went for almond, which it turns out makes for a ridiculously rich coffee, so decadent that I reasoned it must be bad for me, but I wasn't inclined to check.

- Resources: Instagram loves vegan grub. Goes absolutely crackers for it. As do cookbook publishers. If you can't find inspiration for at least a million meals, then you must have your eyes closed.

- Inventiveness: this brief stint of veganism had me cooking again, being inventive. I had to be, really. Dad did go ahead and buy what seemed to be the entire range of M&S vegan ready meals, but we weren't keen. A lot of it was deep-fried, appearing to be a big exercise not in celebrating the taste of vegetables but in trying to hide it. Even sticks of sweet potato had been coated in batter. I love cooking (I still remember my first culinary masterpiece: little cut-out circles of white bread spread with strawberry jam. A five-year-old serving canapés? How precocious), but I stopped for a long time, living on mac and cheese ready meals from the Co-op eaten in the dark. Microwaveable in a few minutes, and the only thing I had confidence in keeping down relatively easily.

- Health: I felt fresh, and righteous. I wasn't waking up dehydrated, I easily had my five a day. I'm gonna live for ever, I thought.
- Animals: you're arguably being a bit kinder to animals when you're not killing, cooking and eating them. Don't quote me on that, but I'm pretty sure of it.

Vegan cons:

- Choice: I looked at the online menu of the nearest pub and the only vegan option out of seventeen choices was a hummus wrap. I'm not keen on sandwiches with the texture of an eclair, so I opted out. This would change if more people were vegan, of course, so technically this problem is partly on me.
- Obsession: I know this has already been over-observed for milquetoast laughs, but you really do find yourself having to say the word 'vegan' quite a lot when trying to be vegan. And every mealtime conversation is taken up by saying, 'It's amazing that you can have a whole meal and none of it is from animals! What I'm eating tastes surprisingly okay!' Perhaps this wears off, but the stereotype suggests not. I never had 'meat eater' as a personality trait, so I don't want 'plant-based' as one either. But this is all a cop-out and obviously so.
- Family: Dad looks quietly depressed during mealtimes.

I may be abandoning veganism, but I've been keeping up with my Spanish lessons. I have to, or else The Owl gets mega-cross. I'm on my way back from Big Tesco with fewer animal products than I'd usually get, and decide to treat myself to an early-morning spin in the car wash at the Shell garage. I'm only two visits away from a free Costa coffee.

'It's only "quick wash" that's available today, is that okay?'

'Oh. Yeah, that's fine, thanks.'

'Do you have a Shell card?'

'Yep, I just scan it in here, do I?' (I know what to do.)

'Any time you're ready.'

'Thanks.'

'Busy night?' the guy asks me.

'Yeah, we had three break-ins to deal with, so . . . bit tired.' For some reason I've spontaneously decided to pretend to be a policeman who's just finished his shift. What . . . the hell?

'Three break-ins?'

'Yeah, that time of year, innit.'

'Right. Do you want a receipt?'

'Nah. Actually, yeah, ta. Have a good one, yeah?' Ah, and now I'm cockney. Textbook.

Back in the car, The Owl has already started to harass me, ordering me to learn my common Spanish phrases. He even arranges for an email to be sent at the same time, but in the third person, like a psycho: 'Hi Robert, keep The Owl happy'. I really don't want to anger him, so I drive home to get to work. I've started to add the words 'you pig' to the end of his orders. 'Time for your Spanish lesson, you pig.' 'Learning Spanish requires daily practice, you pig.' It's a good app for me. I need to be jolted out of idleness, and I'm the teacher's pet, a glutton for reward. Gold stars and likes and retweets nourish me like a Pret Superfood Salad. Every time I complete a little Duolingo sesh, which takes about thirty seconds, rather pathetically it feels like a weight off! I have appeased the bird. Master will be pleased with me. I love it. I pull up to my parents' house and realise I didn't go through the car wash. That sodding owl.

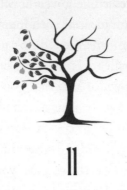

11

Making small changes to everyday things might be key in becoming zen. Three of these everyday things have been big news in weekend supplements lately – veganism, waking up early and tidying. Journalists all across London are regularly writing 1,000 words on one or all of these and summing up with, 'You know what? I just might live like this for ever'. Fifty quid says nearly all of them go back to their normal lives as soon as they've typed the last full stop. Anyway, seeing as I've half-arsed an attempt at veganism, I might as well dip my toe in the other two.

Waking up early, what's it all about? Well, there's a craze amongst highly successful Silicon Valley CEO types and Hollywood people – i.e., 'mega-rich kooks' – of, yep, waking up early. Waking up early and cracking on with all sorts of malarkey. They've discovered that the time when normal people are asleep can also be spent awake, and that this super-early bit of time is the best time, as long as you wake up for it, rather than stay awake until it. Maybe they all just have really uncomfy mattresses, I don't kno~~ ~~ have more money than you can spend, you~~ ~~ hours and minutes.

As I've made quite clear, I'm a sleep fan. Nev~~ ~~ early bird, or a dawn owl, or a sunrise goose, mostly ~~ ~~ I take a long time to stop the cogs and nod off. Always ~~ ~~ skilled at naps, not always so competent at the ol' big sleep (as in kipping soundly through the night, not as in death). Perhaps I need to start catching that worm. My life lacks order. Maybe my jumbled routine leads my mind to panic and indecision. SSRIs help to right the imbalance of chemicals in my brain – I think – the papers recently suggested they do sod all – and having a professional chat every now and then helps me to get on top of my thoughts, but some sort of schedule might go towards further supporting a less nervous break-down-y feeling. I'm reading a book which suggests a richly varied life blossoms from within a framework of repetition and ritual. Have a routine, and mini random adventures will materialise within it. Have a disordered life, and time will just run away with your attempts to cope with it. I've never been proficient at sustaining a healthy routine (though I can sustain an unhealthy one with military precision). Getting up 'well curly' must be inherently good, because people boast about it. 'Did you see the frost this morning?' is code for, 'Were you up as impressively early as me? Because I know you weren't!'

Mark Wahlberg wakes up at 2.30 a.m. He prays at 2.45 a.m., has breakfast at 3.15 a.m. and works out from 3.40 a.m. to 5.15 a.m. He has another meal at 5.30 a.m., a shower at 6 a.m., golf at 7.30 a.m., followed by a snack and then an hour in a cryo chamber. And the day goes on – and on and on – with more snacks and more workouts and snacks and snowers and snacks. He's in bed by 7.30 p.m., ...nably full of snacks and very clean. He seems happy enough. He's certainly more successful than me. I've had days when all I've achieved is turning my pillow to the cold side. From now on I will follow Marky Mark's routine, minus the cryo chamber, whatever one of those is. I imagine it as a sort of lie-down fridge, but I'm probably completely wrong.

It's 2.30 a.m. I went to bed at 9 p.m. and watched *Under the Volcano* with the recently deceased Albert Finney. He was in the film, not in my bed. RIP. I watched it on my iPhone, so my eyes hurt and I think I've crushed my right shoulder. I should order a really long iPhone cable, one that doesn't have to be pinched in a really specific way to convince it to work. I haven't even slept yet but it's time to get up. I'm sleepy, and in fifteen minutes I have to pray to something. I think I'll pray for more sleep.

It's just past 8 a.m. Tip: if you're aiming to get up at 'driving to the airport for the cheapest flight they had' time, don't do your prayers in bed. Prayers, it turns out, unless done in an emergency, are relaxing, and you run the risk of falling asleep until a reasonable hour if you do them on a mattress. Maybe I'll try again tomorrow (reader, I won't). Findings: 1. Waking up early is for the birds; 2. I'm not Mark Wahlberg; 3. If your sleeping pattern ain't broke, don't fix it.

If I can't tidy up my sleep into a neat pattern, surely I can manage it with my piles of stuff? I've always wanted to be clutterless. Tidy house, tidy mind. I keep hold of a hell of a lot of crap. I'll destroy relationships, not look after myself, damage my health, waste buckets of time, burn cash, wash whole chunks of my life down the drain ... but show me a charger and a cable to a phone I had in 2005 and that precious item will be with me for life. What? Throw away this little baggie of spare buttons for a coat I lost on a night out at university, you say? Are you mad? Put it in my coffin when I'm dead.

My wardrobe is traditionally a bomb site. I have bags inside bags inside bags – reach inside any one of them to play 'guess what fruit I used to be'. I take all the receipts out of my wallet and just chuck them in among all the unworn shoes and the hundreds of bits of gym kit that I can no longer fit into. There are wires, cables, books, fondue sets, old toilet bags lined in dried toothpaste, wrapping paper, a yoga mat, suitcases, empty aftershave bottles, full aftershave bottles because they're too nice to use but it's the only thing I can ever think to ask for as a present, photo albums, a cane from when I became obsessed with the TV show *House*, empty picture frames, loose cufflinks, a guitar, huge, empty Selfridges bags (too nice to chuck, aren't they?), spiders, cuddly toy, folders full of old job applications and newspaper clippings, long-dead mobile phones. Oh, and regular old clothes. Amongst other things.

Enter: Marie Kondo. You'll have heard of her. She's the master of organisation. Her philosophy: keep the things that bring you joy, the things that have meaning, and say goodbye to the rest. I want to Marie Kondo my life. Or my cupboards, at least.

I've had a head start on this. When I moved back in with my parents, I just sort of abandoned most of what was in my own wardrobe, and carried an armful of my go-to tops, all the navy ones, to deposit in their spare room wardrobe. I also took three jackets – the same jacket but in navy, maroon and orange, though I only really wear the navy one. Then I bought eight of the same shirt in various colours from Tesco in a succession of two-for-£25 deals, though I've only worn the blue one as of yet. So aside from the Kondo favourite of folding clothes instead of hanging them, which I'm not going to do – hanging is fine, I'm pretty ahead of the game on this adventure. I mean, the wardrobe is half stuffed with expensive Cecil Gee silk shirts that don't fit/suit Dad any more, still smelling of Polo by Ralph Lauren from the big dark green bottle that used to live in his bathroom, but I'm hopeful I'll be able to shrink into those eventually. All I need to do is throw away the tumbleweed of receipts, and I'm done. I'll do that another day.

My wardrobe in my own house is bursting with clobber; I can't say I long for or even remember a single item. I must make sure not to look in it one day or it'll suddenly be the most desirable collection of too-small cheap T-shirts any man has ever seen. Actually, maybe I have Kondo'ed my life, albeit unthinkingly. Perhaps just walking away from mess is as good as purposefully organising it? Something I should probably think about. But anyway, for now I'm a meat-eating, late-rising, messy person, and I think I'm going to stay that way, so my adventures are going to have to accommodate those lifestyle choices.

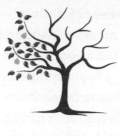

12

'Sir, please, no sliding down the cheese!'

'Really?'

'Sorry, there were some signs up but they've gone. You're not allowed to climb on or slide down the cheese. He'll have to get down.'

I'm at the Cheese & Chilli Festival on a hot late-May day in Bedford, with Mark and my little nephew James dressed in a white T-shirt which says *YEAH* in big black letters. The grass is green, the sky gin clear, cloudless and blue like a screensaver, I'm wearing brand-new pants and the air smells of hot sauce. Oh heavenly day. My first choice of career was cheffing. The day I received my final grade for my three years of English and philosophy lectures, I rang Mum in the morning, two bottles of £3 cava down, to announce that I was going to cook for a living. She said no, you don't wanna do that. Apparently just because at the time I looked like Jamie Oliver (I was even approached by a bloke in a pub who ran a lookalike agency asking if I'd like to be on his books), it did not mean I'd instantly get my own TV show. I'd actually have to learn to cook, and three years of reading Byron does not a decent soufflé make. I thought about accepting the lookalike offer – it would be funny to say to Mum, 'Look, told you I could be Jamie Oliver, albeit a pretend one that nobody has any cause to hire' – deciding it wasn't worth it just for a joke. So, journalism, I'd have a go at that then. It was while I was a journalist for a technology magazine years later that my friend and colleague Joe and I won a burger cook-off at the Taste of London festival. It was one of my proudest achievements and I've always wanted to do something like that again, so I'm here to eat a succession of bastard-hot chilli peppers and win the respect of all of Bedfordshire. It won't have the unpalatable, grotesque greed of stuffing myself like the burger challenge would've done; this is more like martial arts – this is pain control, proper ninja shit.

So yeah, Mark and I have been encouraging James to hurl himself down the large inflatable cartoon wedge of Swiss cheese, as other children have been doing, thinking it part of some wacky playground. I wouldn't mind having a go on it. Growing up with Mark as an older brother, I'm quite used to playtime coming with a risk of death, from testing if a powerful pellet gun would be able to penetrate a heavy leather jacket (thankfully, no), and the thrilling games of 'outrun the frisbee' to the 'sit on my feet and let me launch you' incident. Not to mention when we'd lie on the grass next to each other and use a bow to fire an arrow – a real one – directly up into the sky, so high it would disappear from sight into the glare. Then the countdown, from ten, nine, eight, seven, six, five, four ... the high-pitched scream of the arrow starts to register, buzzing back through the air like a giant mosquito ...

eeeeeeeee ... the temptation to move absolutely unreal ... 'don't move, DON'T MOVE!' ... eeeEEEEEEEEEEE THUD!! Sometimes the arrow would land metres away, burying itself in the turf; once or twice it landed inches away, and once it landed between our heads. We always shut our eyes for protection. Mum didn't like us playing that game. Now that we're being told to move away from this big cheese, we can sort of see why it normally comes with a warning sign: it's twelve foot tall with no steps, barriers or handrails. It would be quite easy to tumble from this slope of mock fromage and end up in a neck brace. Cause of death: fell off a cheese. Embarrassing. We quickly guide James off and away from the cheese and walk across the park towards the large inflatable chilli pepper, which also doesn't have any signs, and climb all over that. It's on its side, so it's only a metre high.

Now that I'm a flexitarian (veggie but with the option to eat meat and dairy whenever I fancy it), I resist sampling any cheese, of which there's a bafflingly small array for what's meant to be 50 per cent a cheese festival, but I do have a souvlaki lamb wrap with some of the chilli sauce we've just purchased. Yes, our mission today is heavily weighted towards the chilli half of things. It's not how I pictured a chilli festival, though; I was expecting it to be more American in style, more of a 'cook-off', like I've seen on *The Simpsons*, with bubbling pots of suicidally spicy, saucy mince to try if you dare, and steaming chilli con carne ladled on to hot dogs slathered in sticky onions, or folded into wraps with grated cheese, guacamole and refried beans, or generously slopped into tin bowls. Instead it's like they've moved the more adventurous section of the Big Tesco condiment aisle outside. There's numerous stands that house various strengths of chilli sauce, jams and oils, that, to the layman, all look pretty similar. At the front of each stand is a tub of lolly sticks, mini squares of tortilla wrap and various sample dishes of orange, bright red and dark red sauce studded with dip marks, going warm in the sunshine. You take part in the same exchange with each stallholder as you make your way around the fest, ruining your tongue as you go:

'Hello there. Have a taste if you fancy.'

'Okay. Hmm, ooh, wow ... that's really nice, actually.'

'Yes, it's not just heat, there's a lot of background flavour as well.'

'Mmm, yeah, tasty, very nice. Cor, the heat grows, doesn't it?'

'Yes, it grows gradually. Try this one, it's a little milder if you don't like too much of a kick.'

'Lovely. Mmm, very nice, yeah, I like that one.'

'Yes, I like that one, too. It's six pounds a bottle or fifteen pounds for three.'

'Right, excellent. Thanks.' Look at all the bottles again, slightly bent down, hands in jacket pockets, look like you're pondering. 'Well ... great stuff, I'll have a look around and I might come back later.'

'Okay then, cheers, see you later.'

'You will!'

The only slightly American thing that happens is when the lady who ordered us off the blow-up cheese jogs through the festival shouting, 'We've got a code red,' into her walkie-talkie. We can only assume someone's either fallen off a gigantic brie or unzipped at a urinal without washing their hands.

I love chilli. Not as much as I used to; I used to be a proper 'chilli head'. It's a very similar sort of personality to the pothead. There's all your different strengths, ridiculous names like 'Satan Blood', 'Grim Reaper' or 'Arse Disaster', or 'Five Finger Death Punch', which I used to get yearly from a chilli shop in Brighton. The names share the same twee zaniness you get with real ale names – ooh, they're cheeky! There's a chilli sauce simply called 'Pain'. And of course there's all your chilli fixings such as badges, T-shirts and tools (cutters, choppers, scrunchers, driers, mini greenhouses . . . you name it. I even have salad tongs shaped like chillis!). On top of that, there's your daredevil element. Who can go the highest? Who can bust through to the alternate capsaicin dimensions? When in the depths of a proper chilli addiction, you think it all must seem rather impressive to the korma fans. How they must be in awe of your sweaty, red, brave face. Hey, they too must wish they look like they're experiencing labour pains. It does feel really good, though, all those pain-suppressing endorphins flooding your veins. And unlike running, you can eat chillis sitting down. Now I'm going grey, I prefer a milder sauce. It's like that phase many go through of trying to prove some kind of point by asking for their steak blue, scoffing at warnings that the particular cut of meat you've chosen will be harder to chew than a flip-flop if taken uncooked. I was this wally. Now I ask for my steak at whatever cooking method renders it most edible. But I still feel that these people, who've chosen to spend the hottest Saturday of the year so far tasting warm condiments in a field, are my people. It's inevitable that here turns out to be the first *Very British Problems* fan I encounter in the wild.

'*Very British Problems*! I love that. I've got the "shorts weather" T-shirt,' he says while pointing at Mark's *Very British Problems* T-shirt from behind his sauce stall.

'Ha, nice one,' Mark says, pointing to me. 'He writes it!'

'Oh yeah? Well ... good stuff,' the fan says, looking confused. He reaches under the table to invite us to try a secret 'round the back' sauce he has with him. The perks of fame. It's called 'God Slayer' (I later find out that the good folks at Wiltshire Chilli responsible for God Slayer, described as 'insanely hot with a strong garlic kick', also offer a limited edition sauce called 'Regret', described as 'insanely hot with a hint of garlic', which is almost twice the heat of God Slayer! These two sauces come in little black bottles which look like poppers, which also have cheeky names, though you wouldn't want to involve either of them in sex. The man wears an evil grin. James looks concerned. We politely decline a taste of God Slayer; we're too old these days for that crazy hybrid stuff.

There seems to be a divide in the chilli world between flavour lovers and heat demons (or burns victims). As we drift around the field we either hear, 'This won't win you any bets, but it tastes nice, I don't see the point in that ridiculously hot stuff that'll just sit in a cupboard for ever', or 'This stuff will blow your face *right* off, go on, taste it, I dare you, you'll die, I promise'. You either have your chilli in your sandwich to give it a bit of sass, or you have your chilli pipetted on to your tongue to render you immobile while your friend films you and laughs.

It's a friendly vibe here. Every trader has such a passion for pepper. How lovely to be so into something. I'm starting to feel sure that that's how you feel drunk without drinking: having a passion. Baudelaire's list of things to get drunk on included wine, poetry and virtue, but what of chilli? I'll look into starting a chilli sauce farm when I get home.

Thankfully we arrived many hours before the chilli competition – it's still ages from starting, and we're all keen to make a move now that the sun is high above and roasting all below. It's a relief not to be involved in the festival beyond being an impartial observer. I was quietly dreading it, and that dread had subtly infected my having a perfectly pleasant time just mooching around. I didn't want the attention. I've already learned this lesson during 'the aborted burger challenge incident' at the diner on the A14, but have since simply disregarded it. Why I always have to con myself into believing I need to be part of the main event to enjoy something properly, I don't know. The eating challenge adventure in January should have taught me this once and for all, but I've ignored that lesson, and nearly, in fact definitely, a little bit, spoilt the day for myself, have purposefully taken some of the shine off. I've had a lovely time just being here among the sauces and the blessed sauce makers, and that's surely adventure enough. A year ago I wasn't capable of walking to get the chilli sauce from the fridge, and here I am engaging in conversations at whole stalls of sauce. It's those extremes again. Rather than be content with a nice day, I had to try to push for an extraordinary day, and then panic myself, bottle it, and all because YOLO/FOMO/Capital-L Living/Insta/ Future Anecdotes demand it. Must stop trying to convince the internet, or myself, or I don't know what, that I'm having a mad one. I'm born to be mild.

It's an easy exchange with a stranger when you're talking about a physical object between you ... in this case, a bottle of sauce. I'm not good at riffing a conversation about nothing. I worry I treat the first ten minutes of chat like I'm being interviewed. I concentrate on giving good answers, and maintaining the correct eye-contact-to-looking-away ratio. I forget to ask anything back. Then I realise I'm doing this and it causes me to stop listening, so I just look rude, or like I'm having a stroke. But today's conversations, with their templates, have been a great success. I'm pleased at how it's gone. I can feel myself welling up ... I've managed to rub chilli sauce in my eyes. We must leave. But first, we have to keep a promise to one of the twenty chilli stand owners we've said we'd revisit with open wallets. Mark walks back and forth between three of the stalls, like a judge at Crufts, then points and strides towards the best in show: Ntsama's. These sauces, we've been told, are hand-prepared from Scotch bonnet chillies and one or two secret ingredients. They're damn tasty. And hot. Tasty and hot. That's all the boxes ticked. My eyes really hurt now. Onwards, to McDonald's, vanilla milkshakes are on me. I wonder if they do a cup large enough to fit a whole head into.

13

Guess where I'm going. No. No, not there. Yes! That's right, I'm off to Spain. Again. I feel it's time to have another run at a solo adventure. Barcelona wasn't particularly a success, but I went too big too soon. And I figured that if I should test my Spanish anywhere, then here, the land of the soaking plain, would be quite suitable. Dress me up in shirts of linen, smother me in Factor 50 (or I can just do that myself) and point me at the nearest Spaniard. I'm not that far on with my Duolingo training, so my plan is to stick to asking for stuff in shops and restaurants, rather than, say, having conversations with local professors about metaphysics, but I feel going these extra miles (in a literal distance sense) will please The Owl.

My app tells me I've saved nearly four grand in the last eight months by just drinking coffees, teas and various flavours of squash, so I'm treating myself to a seat in Club Class. The lounge in Gatwick proves most posh, and a welcome nirvana from the commuter train down here from Huntingdon at 5.30 a.m., where an American man routinely responded to the chat of his English friend by letting out a loud goose-like noise, somewhere between a 'yeah' and a 'honk'.

'Of course they've closed that road now, so ...'

'HEH.'

'You have to go down the back lanes, but it's no trouble ...'

'HEH.'

'Except if you get stuck behind a lorry or something.'

'HEH.'

He alighted at Finsbury Park before I could throw any bread at him.

A British airport lounge basically acts as a huge trough. A place of square leather chairs, USB charging ports and dark wood, where travellers have three little-plate breakfasts in a row, with lashings of all-day booze. Though you have to pretend to be taken off guard by the offer of early drinks. It's just the rules. Pint? Ooh, erm, I shouldn't, but ... yeah, go on then! Glass of bubbles offered on a tray at a wedding? Oh, how lovely, thank you! And so it is in an airport, even though you're helping yourself, you just have the conversation in your own head. 'Well! I didn't expect this, and it's only 7 a.m., but seeing as I'm on me 'olidays!' There'd be revolt if it wasn't provided.

I help myself to a morning full-fat Coke. I feel guilty. Feels like stealing! It's that immediate, short-lived type of guilt, the sort I feel when I'm forced to press the button to stop traffic at a pelican crossing. Every time they bring out a fresh tray of bacon sandwiches on a trolley, which is the top culinary prize this morning, of most mornings, a group of men rise, leaving their cheek prints in the square, plump leather chairs and gather, like a *Top Gear* studio audience, around the person tonging the sandwiches into place at the counter. I am one of these men. Here we huddle and hop like tall, tubby penguins sharing warmth, waiting for the bacon-bringer to leave, whereby we dart off our marks like F1 cars – *GO GO GO!* – towards the smallest, most distinctively average bacon sandwiches ever to be wheeled into a room. A single rasher folded in half inside a mini ciabatta, with white bowls of ketchup and brown sauce on the side. Some bloke dressed in camouflage-patterned shorts and matching tight camo T-shirt takes three in one giant paw! Is that allowed? I take (I just take it! Nobody stops me, like they do in the shops!) a water, a flapjack and a banana. Not that I plan to eat the banana any time soon: I find it bad manners to eat most fruits, especially the peelable sort, in front of strangers. I remember one of my bosses telling me in my appraisal why I wouldn't be getting a pay rise for another year, despite being handed a more senior role, while he peeled an obscenely large orange. The small meeting room smelled strongly of citrus. He was dripping juice all over himself and the table. I think about it only three or four times a day now. I stuff the loot in my bag. This is what it must be like to be a celebrity. I'd be quite happy to just have a holiday in this lounge, to be honest.

Club Class on this flight to Alicante seems to involve sitting further up the plane and getting a menu with a choice of three meals, two of which – chicken salad and salmon penne – aren't available. Beef stew it is, then, which is what I'd decided on anyway, my appetite not in any way diminished from five bacon sandwiches taken only an hour ago. Maybe the brain encourages us to eat so much when travelling in case we crash in the mountains and want to last at least a few days before we start to chew each other. Maybe I'm just greedy.

To signify you're in Club Class, there's a curtain between

you and the rest of the plane behind. I'm in the last row of Club Class – there's only four or five rows – and this curtain gets accidentally pulled over my head, so for a brief moment, my body is enjoying the luxury of the front of the plane, but my face is not. The family behind me find this hilarious. A happy young woman boards, one of the final few through the cabin door, and scans the overhead bins (why bins?). I know what's going to happen before it inevitably does. She sees what probably looks like an empty space in the locker above me. Upon getting closer and going on tiptoes, she'd see this locker actually contains my rucksack. She apparently sees this not as a shame, but as a challenge. Taking her giant rose-gold metal case, covered in funny stickers, she rams my poor bag, then rams it again, and again, and again, with such sustained savagery you'd think it contained a tiny man who she'd been paid to put in a coma. I sit and massage my temples with stiff fingers (my fingers, though someone else's would be nice; I should get a head massage at some point) and try not to contemplate just how much irreversible damage she's doing to my banana.

People nervously enquire about how many little miniature bottles of gin they're allowed, the acceptable midday spirit, smiling as they're plonked on their trays, reminding me of when I broke into the locked cupboard of my parents' min-iatures collection when I was eight and downed a load of weird spirits, apparently taking a particular shine to cherry brandy. I can't remember it. Mark found me unconscious on the bathroom floor. I only remember waking up in intensive care a few days later, with a doctor standing over me saying, 'You little tinker.' Nearly snuffed it, I'm told.

The flight is proving relatively uneventful, which is my

preferred type of aeroplane experience, when, over Madrid, where the Champions League Final is due to take place tomorrow, the lady a few rows in front of me dies. Her husband, who looks like Claude Littner, Lord Sugar's adviser on *The Apprentice*, frantically waves his hands to beckon someone, anyone. For a second I think he's just really keen for some complimentary nuts, but each rising level of panic leapfrogs the last with great speed until a dead end of pure fear finally freezes him into stillness. Nowhere to run. Nowhere to hide. Medical machines and oxygen masks are wrenched from lockers. 'Madam, can you hear me?' is said, then shouted, then shouted again; people start to remove their headphones and pop their heads (mostly baseball-capped heads – there always seems to be a higher than average concentration of baseball caps on planes) over their seats. It looks like a human game of whack-a-mole. The dead wife's husband, now half standing, stupidly trapped by the overhead locker above his window seat, darts his eyes around for a door to a reality where this isn't happening to her and to him. To them. How many of us, feeling guilty for being unable to help, wonder if the plane will have to divert? What happens if someone dies on a plane? Do they just leave them in their seat? Do they drag them (feet first?) to the galley? Maybe there's a special cupboard. I wish I wasn't thinking this. Surely she hasn't just died, that would be ridiculous, it would ... Oh, she's awake. Hang on, is she? Yep, she is. Turns out she'd enjoyed some/ quite a bit of white wine for breakfast and had drifted off with her eyes open ('this has happened before'), becoming visibly alive again after what must have been an entire minute. After a few chuckles of pure relief, the husband makes sure to have a jokey, apologetic chat to us all one by one before we all pop our headphones on again and go back to thinking about all sorts.

Before Spain, I'd tried to make a head start on my tan. I'm a new potato that requires some par-boiling, so on Mum's recommendation I visited the stand-up 'Collatan' tanning booth at Salon 41, nestled between Thelma's Flowers and The Grand Piano café. Opposite Flameboyant, which sells stoves and fireplaces. Mum had told me, 'It does blemishes, it does anxiety, it does inflammation, it does depression, it's a wonderful machine.' Despite receiving treatment for skin cancer over the past twenty years, Mum has never fallen out of love with UV. On my arrival I was shown through the salon by a lady, who told me shyly it was her first day, so she was a bit nervous to be giving instructions. Relieved to find she hadn't accidentally turned the toaster settings up too high, I exited the bronzing coffin, which plays loud dance music, presumably in case the fierce red light and jet engine noise lulls you to slumber, after three minutes looking and feeling exactly the same, my giblets intact and not defrosted in the slightest. I suppose it's not an instant thing. I mustn't become addicted to it, mustn't become the Red Man of Godmanchester.

I go a further three times over the next week, and also get my toenail gelled. In my twenties I was rocking out on a Les Paul electric guitar when the strap broke, sending the full weight of the thing on to my big toe. I whipped my right sock off and blood sprayed everywhere. I knew at that very moment I wouldn't ever be a rock star. That wasn't even the most painful bit – that was reserved for casualty, where they stitched up my nail bed, which left a permanent crack down the middle. The gel helps it stay firmly together as one nearly normal nail. I was covering Crufts for *Your Dog Magazine* the day after toe-gate, for the whole weekend, so could be seen among the retrievers and terriers, hobbling around in one sandal with a dictaphone. Ben Fogle said no when I asked him for an interview, and I mention it every time he comes on the telly. It was nice, though, having my one nail done. Relaxing. I might go back and ask for the works. Maybe pampering can be my thing. I've written *Bathe in milk?* in my notebook, which will mystify me when I read it in about a year.

I landed in Alicante about two hours ago. Now I'm in Teluada, between Valencia and Benidorm, shivering at the *queso* counter of a freezing Pepe La Sal *supermercado*. Not only is it cold but it's so clean, like a futuristic hospital. Like Princeton-Plainsboro Teaching Hospital in *House*. You could probably perform an appendectomy on the floor and not have to worry about infection. Between the airport and here, I've found no need to speak Spanish, or in fact any language at all. There's certainly no real need to speak in this supermarket, or in any supermarket now I think about it. I walk up to the milk section, pick up a carton of milk and put the milk in my basket. I do the same with other items. This is an anti-climax. I forgot that in most shops you don't have to actually do much asking, it's mostly just picking up what you need. Aha! Cheese counter! Here's my chance ... play it cool, Trig, play it cool ...

'*Hola.*'

'*Hola!* Erm ... *una* ... slice ... roquefort, *por favor?*'

'Roquefort, yes, this piece?'

'*Si*, that's lovely, *gracias.*'

'Anything else for you?'

'No, that's great. *Gracias.*'

'*Gracias, adios.*'

'Cheers.'

Well, that was pathetic. I could've done so much better than that. I've trained hard, but I lost my nerve (what nerve?). I feel like punching the huge pig leg in front of me. Whatever would The Owl think? I imagine him stomping around, furious, like Alan Rickman as the Sheriff of Nottingham. He's going to carve my heart out with a spoon.

'Shit!' I blurt by means of apology as I step back into someone's trolley. 'No worries,' says the lady in the oversized Liverpool shirt. '*Pardon,*' I offer, in a French accent. I should leave. I pay for my milk, roquefort, chorizo slices, ham crisps, jelly sweets, five litres of *agua*, bread, coleslaw, large jar of gherkins, hot sauce and mint ice cream and drive to the Airbnb, where I can't work out how to watch the football. People from all over the world have flooded to Spain by car, boat, bike and aeroplane to watch the biggest match of the year in the stadium and surrounding streets. I've come to the country for no reason other than to buy milk, and I can't work out how to watch the match on the telly. I end up listening to it on Radio 5 while eating coleslaw that doesn't taste at all like the coleslaw back home. Definitely should've stayed in the airport lounge. I could be on my hundredth free Coke by now. I could've grown a beard and become fat with bacon rolls. That would be my thing; I'd become known for it. I'd wear a big red smock and people would call me Airport Santa. 'He never goes anywhere, he just sits in that corner, jiggling his belly like a bowlful of jelly . . . NO, DON'T APPROACH HIM!' I wish I knew what I'm doing. How many years is 'I'm in a bit of a weird place at the minute' meant to last?

I don't know whether to be pleased with myself because in

this, the year of adventure, I'm travelling on planes to faraway lands (okay, mostly Spain) more than I was going through my front door not too long ago. Or if I should feel disappointed because I'm frittering money away and stamping around leaving big carbon footprints with the net result of sitting in bedrooms on my own, abroad. Shall I change tack, or keep at the travel? I just don't know. I'm tired of my own imagination, or lack thereof, and annoyed at myself for being so bloody lame. I should try exploring Britain a little more.

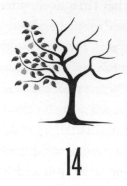

14

I've always wanted a sea view. Always love to see the ocean. Who doesn't? I've been landlocked for a long time – time to see the sea. They say people are generally happier when they're by water. Unless they're drowning. Where's a good, big bit of water? The internet suggests Blackpool. Sounds adventurous. Yes, I'll go on a jolly boys' outing on my own, that'll be good.

If only it was sunny. It's clammy. It's June and it's a heavy grey Monday. The sky has been colour-matched in B&Q with John Humphrys. Actually I think it might have been John Humphrys' 'Regret' we chose for the living room walls. The A1 is grey. England seems to be stored inside a complimentary hot towel today. I pass by Retford, where I got badly sunburned while fishing for carp as a student and earned the nickname Lobster Rob, having to go to Sainsbury's before a party later that night, where a checkout girl helped apply thick, cheap, dark foundation to my face, so rather than just looking like a sunburned man I looked like one who'd fallen in some Ronseal. Those were the days, when I went to parties all sizzled, rather than now, where I visit B&Q for fun and spend half the day worrying I might be deficient in the B vitamins. I turn left somewhere around Leeds, onto the M62. Crossing over the River Ribble, which I can't help but think of as being said by Rowan Atkinson, I start to wonder, again, what I'm doing, with life in general. But mostly on my journey I feel nothing at all; I can't decide whether that's welcome, or lucky, or a shame, and I don't try to work it out for too long. All is fine when you're driving. I do however feel a little like this is my 'Alan Partridge driving to Dundee in bare feet' moment. Perhaps it's a mistake for me to have pathetic comedy characters as heroes.

Blindly following Google Maps causes none of the 'and then I ended up in a field on a cliff full of tigers!' stories you occasionally see in the papers, which I'm sure are either bollocks or, if not, should get the drivers involved banned from operating a car. A final right turn takes me along the promenade, past the giant mirrorball, which today has nothing to reflect. The Headlands Hotel looks to be boarded up, but as I do an overly dramatic five-point turn after deciding that reverse parking would be best in this large, empty car park, my tyres crackling over the fine grey gravel like a giant bowl of Rice Krispies, I spot the receptionist watching me through the window. Open for business, then. Good stuff. It's a small, pretty hotel with a too-small revolving door. There should be size limits for revolving doors. This one seems to be the size of a NutriBullet. Inside all looks perfectly pleasant, but my chest has tightened, my head has clouded and I now have an overwhelming desire to drive back home. But then, like rain, I expected that.

'Hello, checking in?' says the smiling woman behind reception, who is the only staff member I see during my stay. She's friendly and calming. She has large eyes, in a nice way, not in a medical problem way. 'I was just imagining your door filled up with frozen fruit,' my mind says, which creates a good three seconds before I actually reply, 'Yes, please. Temple. Robert Temple.' Steady on, 007.

'Right, let's have a look.' She scans a folder. 'I can actually put you in a larger room, we're not full.'

She leads me to a room upstairs, hands me the key and leaves me to it. There's a sea view, a slight smell of cigarettes, which I suppose you can never truly get rid of when an old place is 90 per cent carpet (and to be honest, I might have just been imagining the scent), a duvet screwed up on the floor, wet towels in the bath and a half-full cup of tea. After I've put six shirts on un-stealable hangers, of which I'll wear one – the navy one – I decide that, actually, I should probably say something about the state of the place. I was prepared to just make the bed myself, but then started to worry that the last occupant might have had a lot of loose back hair, or a hatred of pyjamas and pants coupled with a lackadaisical attitude to waist-down hygiene and a penchant for sitting on pillows.

'Oh no, I'm so sorry about that, they must have missed it off the rota. I'll move you to another room, let me just have a look. Yes, here we are.'

Handed another key, I go back up two flights to my first room to pack my shirts, tidy up a bit, lock the door behind me, travel down one flight of stairs to a tidy room, identical in layout, with a view of what I'm certain must be the same sea, and rehang my shirts. Then I lie down on the bed, shoes still on but feet hanging off the end of the mattress. I must not under any circumstances just stay in this position until it's time to go home. I must not close my eyes. *Do not waste this day*. Could just lie here, though, I suppose. Who would know? No. This is going to require a countdown. Focus. Five, four, three, two, one, go. Ready for launch. Up you get! Any second now. Five, four, three, two, one, NOW! GO! Any second now, I'll get up. Oh, just get up, you lazy berk. I'm up! I'm on the move. Locking the door, I walk away, then walk back to check I've locked the door (I have), then bounce back to reception to hand back the old key. 'See you later!' Whoosh, I'm spinning in the revolving door like a badly out-of-shape Clark Kent trying to change into his work clothes, and then out into sunny Blackpool. I'm free. Right, let's look at the map ... about an hour's walk to Blackpool Tower, certainly a good chance for some exercise, a brisk traipse to town will be sure to clear my head. Fantastic. I get straight on a tram.

'Can I have a day ticket, please,' I say, handing over a crisp rectangle of paper money.

'Ooh, you haven't got the exact change, have you?' queries the short, friendly, uniformed young man who looks like an extra in *Quadrophenia* getting through his day job before whacking on a parka and scootering home to pin up newspaper clippings about Keith Moon above his bed.

'No, sorry, I don't think so.'

'First job on a Monday, you see, always the one where someone gives you a fifty-pound note and expects change,' he chuckles, holding the £10 note I gave him.

'Sorry about this,' I say, gripping onto the handrail in case we suddenly start moving, while he opens up a bag stuffed to the brim with coins, enough change to fill Scrooge McDuck's swimming pool.

'Don't worry about it, sir,' he says, handing me the exact amount required. 'Always happens. Enjoy yourself.'

There is no queue at the payment desk at the base of the Blackpool Tower, which is not to say there's not plenty of customers trying to be served, it's just that there's nothing I'd refer to as a queue. There's that same musty carpet smell that seems to be everywhere, however. Perhaps it's me. People (it's always people, isn't it?) are milling around, pretending they've never heard of or imagined the concept of a queue in their lives. They all adopt expressions of 'oh, do we just ... walk to the front? I guess that's the system ...' Their wide-eyed innocence doesn't fool me, and I let them know this by silently exploding with rage inside my own head while keeping an expression of a bored husband staring out across Debenhams.

A young couple with a baby head past me, in my queue of one, straight to the desk, enquire about going up the tower, are told they can go up the tower if they want, are then informed of the prices of going up the tower, and take that moment to stand at the desk and have a long discussion with each other about whether they're interested in going up a tower today. They even consult the baby. After five years of deliberation, they decide not to go up the tower, instead enquiring if it'd be okay to GO UP THE TOWER ANOTHER DAY? Yes, the lady manning the till replies; of course it fucking is. How I'd love it if she actually said this. I am one limp burger away from going Michael Douglas, except without the guns. I tell myself to stop being so angry, stop trying to bend the world to you. Nobody asked you to come here. Maybe I'm doing it on purpose because I think I'm the VBP man with the bowler hat from the book. No, no, I am really like this, unfortunately. I'm about to break my own neck by tensing too much. Calm down. By the time I'm paying for my ticket, I have already ruined the experience for myself. Anxiety causes me to get so quietly wound up because I'm constantly trying to communicate my dissatisfaction with a situation by thinking about it really intensely, and then getting pissed off, that nobody can hear what I'm not saying.

I'm directed towards the worst lift in the world. It reminds me of those fitting rooms you get in Sports Direct, or holiday resort gift shops. The sort that are really tiny storage areas rather than fitting rooms, in which someone has placed a ripped leather stool and no hooks. It takes me a while to get in this lift. The first time it opens, a couple peer out the door, as if considering whether it's safe to step from a lunar module without risking floating off into space for ever. Seemingly terrified, they ask nobody in particular, 'Is this Ground? Ground? Is this Ground?' Did you press G, I wonder? Is the digital screen showing a big red G? Have you come from above? Does this look clearly like the lobby where you presumably entered, unless you somehow started your experience of the Blackpool Tower at the summit? Before I could say yes, this is G, the doors begin to close and the couple visibly panic to a degree that I suspect their lives flash before their eyes and *ding*, off they pop, back skywards. The next time the lift door opens on G, it is empty. I don't see that couple again.

The tiny lift takes you not to the top of the tower, but to a 3D cinema experience all about Blackpool. Well, technically it's 4D, because at one point some sort of dandruff sprays out, like someone has come up behind me and blown the icing off a cake. But mostly it's just the experience of being startled by various things you wouldn't want to have smacking you in the face in real life appearing to smack you in the face. Blackpool looks really nice in the film. There's only one other person in the cinema, which is strange considering the number of people buying tickets downstairs: a white man with blond dreadlocks who, for the duration of the film, wears his 3D glasses not over his eyes, but propped up on top of his head. Strange thing to do, I think, as I give myself whiplash flinching at an animated bird suddenly spearing me through my forehead. After this, it's up to the tower top proper in a big fancy glass lift, in which a tiny, nervous young woman, I guess a student, asks if myself and Dreadlocks have enjoyed the tower so far.

'Yeah, it's been cool, you know?' he says, in an accent like mine: plain. 'Although I'm not really here for the tower, you know?' No, no idea. But at least he speaks. I can't get any words out. When people tell me I'm quiet I tend to say, 'Am I? Sorry. I don't mean to be.' Being quiet unsettles people, makes them think something's wrong; that you're not having a good time, or that they're annoying you. 'You're quiet,' is said because your timidity is causing yours and their insecurities to clash and bind together. You rarely get people saying, 'You're loud,' to a noisy person, because noise is easier to deal with than quiet. Noise stops everyone thinking too much. Silence is hard work. I never tell people they're loud. Perhaps because I'm quiet. If I'm at a group meal and someone says, 'You're quiet,' to me, it feels like the entire world has just turned its eyes towards my chair and demanded, 'Speech!' I sit there thinking, 'Oh, just speak, you moron, get over yourself, nobody cares, in fact you'd make it a lot more comfortable for everyone if you just said ... well, *anything*!' All this is going through my head, instead of words coming out of it. While I'm buttering my bread, staring into space, I'm actually writing 'Why I'm Not Speaking – a thesis, by Rob Temple, for Rob Temple' in my head. Again. This thought process, which is easily mistaken for daydreaming, is what caused my biology teacher in senior school, Mr Earl, to write, 'I feel I need to place a bomb under his seat to shock him from his reverie', in my report card.

Of course, sometimes I am simply staring into space, my mind as blank as my 2018 diary. This usually happens when I'm asked a simple question, such as when Richard Bacon interviewed me live (millions of listeners. Christ) on Radio 1, him in a studio, me in a pissy phone box on Bedford Hill in Balham. My phone conked out, so I had to run to the box in swimming trunks and a vest, full of cider. 'So, tell us about *Very British Problems!*' Erm ... well ... it's ... erm ... hello? Can you hear me? Erm ...' I asked Juliet how I'd done once Richard Bacon had cut me off. 'It was good, very on-brand,' she replied. 'The only thing is you forgot to mention the book.'

I zone back in to the sound of the lift lady telling us about the tower, about how the very top is closed (first mention of this since paying and entering the building), and that the glass floor can withstand five tons, so we should feel free to have a good jump about on it. And then the doors open at very nearly the top of the tower. There's a handful of others facing large windows. And then ... I see it. I see what they're seeing. It's breathtaking. I've looked up in wonder at the ceiling of the Sistine Chapel; I've sipped a glass of hot wine while staring at the Northern Lights; I've seen it rain so hard the drains became clogged up with hay and we tried to clear it by ramming a big stick into the grate but the stick just broke off and clogged the drain even more ... but nothing prepares you for this: endless grey as far as the eye can see. The windows might as well be painted grey. I've travelled over four hours and paid to be thrust into the sky via two lifts for the experience of being in an out-of-control steam room. I can't help but feel it's fantastic. Much better than a view, really. I can imagine a view, or look on Google, but this just makes me LOL inside. How wonderfully typical. So very-bloody-British. And by the way, people get really freaked out when you do have a jump about on a really high-up glass floor. One woman shrieks.

There's a bar up here. Dreadlocks orders a gin and tonic, and not once do I see him face the 360-degree windows. What's the point, I suppose. Hang on, he wasn't into the 4D experience either. Surely he's not just here for a drink? I go back down again: £27 all in. This also included a ticket to Sea Life (which I imagine 'doesn't have any big fish today'), but I'm not in the mood for marine life, so for a short while I unsuccessfully try to give the ticket away outside the tower. I think I have a 'don't accept fish tickets from this man' vibe, due to my cross face and uncomfortable mumbling. I consider going to Blackpool Pleasure Beach to try to feel some excitement on the Big Dipper, but it's closed. Teatime is spent in a nice Pizza Express, a dependable friend more than a restaurant, where I have the pizza I always have, a rectangular spicy one. Then I sit in a bar for enough time to see a frowzy fella with faded blue jeans and a beer belly under a baggy white short-sleeve shirt dancing on his own to 'Johnny B. Goode'. I think he might have had a few ales. In fact, everyone in Blackpool seems to have had a few ales, apart from me. He puts his foot on the stage one too many times and gets violently dragged out by two giants in black coats, both more rhino than man. Right, think I'll call it a night. Taxi! The cab driver spends the journey telling me Blackpool has changed. He doesn't suggest how it's changed or why, just keeps repeating.

'Blackpool, it's changed, you know?'

'No? How?'

'You know, everyone knows Blackpool, you know? They used to come here ... now people come here, and it's not the same, it's changed ... you know?'

'Oh, right, yeah. That's a shame.'

'Yeah, it's not the same, man, not the same at all.'

'Not the same as it was?'

'Exactly! Exactly.'

I'm seated for breakfast. I've said that a pot of tea would be lovely, and just as I'm off to visit the glass jugs on the neatly set up side table, to choose between a small tumbler of red, orange or yellow (or maybe a mix of all of them! Whoa there!) an elderly gentleman with fluffy white candyfloss hair, and puffy hands that look like unevenly toasted pita bread, raises a piece of dripping buttery toast, like a referee giving me a casual yellow card for celebrating a goal by taking my shirt off (what's the deal with that celebration, anyway?), and wishes me a good morning. 'Thank you, same to you. Looks like it's brightening up,' I trill, though it looks like it's getting darker, if anything. 'Up to much today?' I enquire. He doesn't hear me, so, like a man who's just waved at someone who's waving at someone behind him, I slowly turn my head back to my table and fiddle with my knife and fork with an inane, wilting, wasted polite smile on my chops.

'Okay, here we go, one full English, can I get you anything else?' No, that's lovely, thanks. It's a handsome breakfast – Gemma and I once heard someone describe their breakfast as 'double 'andsome', the highest of all breakfast praise – all neat and tidy on the big white plate, arranged with unfussy finesse. 'Quite possible! Quite possible!' the elderly man chuckles, about a minute too late. 'Fingers crossed!' I reply, as fried egg slips off my fork on to the lap of my light pink shorts. Marvellous. The lady at the table to the right of us, also no spring chicken, requests her bacon 'very well done' and her fried egg 'quite medium'. Then, once our hostess has taken that down on her pad and returned to the kitchen, the elderly lady tells her younger companion (daughter, I decide) that she always buys 'real bacon', which she stores in a shoe-box in the cupboard, rather than not in a shoebox and in the fridge. Although the large room we're dining in, which feels to me a bit like it's on a ferry, is half-empty, we're all sat within touching distance of each other. Everyone with someone to talk to does so in those stilted conversations about nothing that mean they know everyone can hear. Waiting room chat. The breakfast is hot and tasty.

Pacing around my room, tapping my pockets every five minutes, 'wallet, phone, keys, headphones', I wait until checkout time. Wallet, phone, keys, headphones. I clean the two mugs on my bedside table, but then worry they might be mistaken for mugs that haven't been used, so I fill them both with water. Wallet, phone, keys, headphones. Checkout time is taking ages. Once I've removed myself from the hotel, I chuck my mini suitcase into the boot of the car and venture back into the bustling bit of Blackpool, to a shop, I forget the name, to look for some sort of souvenir. I have a stick of rock in mind. There's a birthday coming up soon, too, so I need to sniff a load of scented candles. I've given a decent chunk of my life to standing in shops sniffing scented candles. Trying to find an acceptable smell, usually before too much of my lunch hour runs out. Magnolia and Sea Balm, Lavender and Fog, Sand et Time, Summer Snow, Myrrh and Blood, Vinegar and Piss ... below £30 and they usually smell like Glade, so you really have to hunt. A lady with a pram is encroaching on my sniffing zone. She wants to sniff where I'm sniffing. She wants to also work out, 'Does this smell say I value my friend?' I decide to just abandon the whole plan because I'm sweating and there's a man in a suit in front of me who looks like a door-to-door salesman from 1950s America down on his luck, tie loosened and hair messily slicked back, attempting to angrily return a life-size inflatable Spider-Man because it's 'not what I expected at all'. Something tells me he won't be quickly appeased.

Rock and candles postponed, it's time to head back to the hotel car park. Driving away from Blackpool in the thunder, I feel simply tired. Perhaps a bit confused, but no more than usual. Quite alone, which is understandable, I suppose, as I'm on my own. I used to think I was good at being alone, but I'm absolutely pants at it. I was only good at being alone when I had a choice. Need to work out how to 'be here now' but without having to read a book about it ... will probably make a mental note to make a physical note of this thought later. I'd love a drink but I don't want to come out in hospitals. A roadside Greggs appears, as if it's a mirage. That's the ticket! I like Greggs. We all like Greggs. KEEP CALM AND PLOUGH ON, reads a large poster on the wall. Yes, that's the spirit. Necessary, too, as it's another three hours back to Godmanchester. I'm grateful to Greggs for the pep.

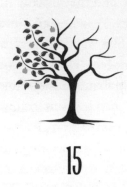

15

When you're climbing Everest, leave your ego at home. Don't take negativity up with you, else She'll be grumpy right back at ya. You have to respect the mountain – you're not deciding to climb Her, She's allowing you to, for you assail in Her grace. This is the kind of bonkers thing you read in books about hauling yourself up monstrous great rocks. I decided I needed to put a bit more effort in if I were to see a glorious sea view, a decision which now finds me halfway up to the Torre Vigia Cap d'Or. Yes, Spain again. I thought about somewhere else, but you know where you are with Spain. You're in Spain. And my parents are here too. Welcome to another adventure with stabilisers with your armbanded hero.

The trek to the watchtower, known locally as the pepper pot, is me and Dad's own Everest. Sure, it's not quite as taxing as a mountain – phrases highlighted about the endeavour on TripAdvisor include 'nice walk', 'take care' and 'wear trainers' – but he's seventy-one and I'm lazy, so. Despite the friendly online recommendations towards wearing proper shoes, Dad goes for sandals. Packing a rucksack with a bottle of water, a pack of Maltesers (soon to become a parcel of brown goo) and a new pencil (I don't know why), we set off, brave warriors, towards our base camp (the beach). It's so warm in the midday sun that even mad dogs have decided to stay indoors. We pass an ice cream board, standing outside a little café, and I immediately get a craving for a pink foot lolly.

Dad wears the expression of a man who'd really rather be lying on a sunbed doing his Codeword puzzles, not just now but always. You can tell by all the moaning about going that he doesn't want to go. But we'd read that it only takes twenty minutes to get up there, so all being well we'd be making our push on the summit by 11.30 a.m. and back well in time for lunch. Mum's promised cheese and ham toasties, which she does in the microwave so one half's damp and floppy. It's how they like them. We don't chat much as we wind our way up the hot, steep slopes, past villas of various styles and states of repair that climb high up the hills of El Portet. It's that level of steep where you have to lunge with your hands on your thighs instead of stepping. 'Madonna used to have a place here, apparently,' Dad tells me. 'I know, I remember you saying.' After six or seven minutes we go through a fence, swapping road for dusty dirt track, which signifies the start of the climb proper, which I'll refer to as The Death Zone. There's a sign: 'Torre Vigia Cap D'or 805 m/30'. The only way now . . . is up. Unless we turn round and go back down again.

'Bloody hell, you can see why they say to wear shoes. It's a bit treacherous,' says Dad, a man so sensible and cautious that we still all talk about the time he jumped into a swimming pool on holiday rather than use the steps. My eyes are stinging quite a bit from Factor 50 and sweat mingling and dripping through my eyelashes. A family comes into sight on their way down. Two women, one man and three girls no older than ten, in beachwear and flip-flops. The man's shoulders and nose glow medium rare. Mum should toast the sandwiches on him.

'You can see why they tell you to wear shoes,' one of the women says, breathless and chuckling.

'I was just saying!' Dad chuckles. Like me he reserves his laughter for strangers.

'*Hola*,' I offer, even though these legends sound like they're also from Peterborough.

'Hiya, we got a bit lost, we've turned back.'

'Is it up there?' Dad asks.

'Oh yeah, it's definitely up there. There's signs and stuff. Apparently you just keep going up but we went wrong somewhere,' pants the man. He turns and points. 'But it's up there.' It certainly is. We can all see it.

'*Gracias*.'

We clamber on.

'I'm going to take a picture.'

'Don't go near the edge, Robert!'

'It's fine.'

'No, come on, get back.'

'It's okay, I'd go to the edge if I was on my own.'

'No, no no no, NO. Don't. Come on, don't be silly. Taking a picture from here is fine. Come on. Mum wouldn't like it.'

Dad talks a lot about Mum on the climb. How she'd 'have a fit' being up here, how she wouldn't like it at all. Over the next ten or so minutes the path becomes dustier, drier, yellower; I become sweatier. The sea becomes further away, as you'd expect. I'm a short distance ahead, leading the big push. The summit appears all of a sudden, like they tend to. About half a minute later, Dad's salt-and-pepper locks come into view over a ridge, a curious badger seeking shade.

'Well, Dad, first words on reaching the summit?'

'Thank god we're here.'

We pause for a few seconds to stare at the sparkling ('*con gas*') sea and cloudless (looking at you, Blackpool) pale blue sky with expressions that say, 'Yup, that's the sea and sky all right.' We pass a bottle between us, taking turns to sip *agua*, then ring Mum to let her know we're safe. No answer. 'Here, Dad, give me your sandals. You can have my trainers, they're much comfier.' 'No, no, it's fine.' 'Honestly, you can't walk down in those things, you'll fall off the edge.' Dad sits on a rock while I help him on with my trainer socks, which feels weird. The socks are quite sweaty by now and go on with a bit of a struggle. I feel a lot more jelly-legged in the sandals. We're both size ten and these seem to be at least size seventeen. But he's steadier in my trainers, which is the main thing.

'You should wear proper shoes next time.'

'Ha ha . . next time?!'

'Yeah! Just think, now you can sit on the beach and look up and think, "I climbed that!"'

'What, when I'm in my wheelchair, you mean?'

'I can push you up and you can freewheel to the bottom.'

'Look, stop nattering and concentrate, it's a long way down.'

'We're mountain goats.'

'Hmm. I don't know about that.'

Tumbling down the mountainside we go, scrambling occasionally, but mostly just thudding, clomping, hopping. Eventually, when things start to even out, Dad becomes chattier.

'That wasn't too bad, I suppose.'

'Not many people of seventy would be ...'

'Seventy-one.'

'Yeah, not many people of seventy-one would be going up and down something like that, you know, Dad. You've done well.'

'Mum wouldn't like it.'

They've both been in such good shape for as long as I've known them (all my life, really), and still look so youthful, that I forget they're what you could call 'getting on a little' now. Mum's joints give her a lot of pain. I catch their stoic fears of degeneration in glimpses, each one a little ice pick to the heart. I hope their future together stretches far into the distance.

Dad's dad died at forty-seven, a heart attack slumping him over his desk in the office they shared. Dad witnessed it from his own desk, aged only nineteen at the time. Then it was up to him to run the business and look after his siblings and mother. It was 1969, just before the moon landing. They'd been following it keenly together. The fiftieth anniversary of that one small step is coming up; no doubt Dad and I will watch all the tributes to it on telly. Anyway, here he is, in his eighth decade, trotting up to sky-high pepper pots. He's bone dry, as well. My back looks like I've been hosepiped. I'm not sure why, but he gets on to talking about Florida.

'We went there in 1981. This was before they'd built the Epcot Center, I think. We didn't go for long, Mum said you don't need more than a day at a funfair. You hadn't been born then ...'

'I know.'

'You were born in 1983.'

We get back to the villa, seven thousand steps and a few dozen mosquito bites later, where Dad searches every room until he finds Mum standing outside by the balustrade, taking a break from watering plants to monitor the building work going on next door. He can't wait to start telling her all about his adventure, as he's always done.

16

Perhaps it's the coffee. I shouldn't drink it. The withdrawal started to kick in from not Instagramming anything at all for over two days, so I dashed into Costa to photograph a cortado. Then, reluctantly, I drank it. Not too keen on hot drinks, as a rule. Caffeine really gets to work on me quickly; by the time I was out the door and back on to Huntingdon High Street I was buzzing my moobs off. I'm still on a high now as I walk across the footbridge and back into Godmanchester, and have just developed a powerful urge to have a go at some 'classic banter'. I'm not skilled at vocal bantz. I can't 'hold court' – I'm not a 'cheeky chappie'. I've never for a second been in danger of being described as possessing 'joie de vivre', which I'm okay about, really, because anyone who has ever self-identified as having joie de vivre, or as a 'bon viveur', for that matter, has annoyed me deeply. Not many people know that bon viveur is actually an acronym for 'bellowing omnivorous nuisance, versed in verbal ejaculation, usually rat-arsed'. One of my (many) worst nightmares takes the form of the dreaded wedding table plan. The exhaustion of finding out the names of a group of strangers that you'll be required to jest with over the next two hours, immediately after you've tried to convince them that your job is 'boring, really'. Even if I was an astronaut about to head to Mars in a rocket I'd built myself, I'd still say, 'Yeah, it's all right, pays the bills. It's not as fun as it sounds, though ... in fact it's pants.' Then they might reply that it does sound pants and I'd feel aggrieved. Why can't weddings be silent affairs? It's not really other people, of course, it's me. I'm a misery guts, seeing the worst wherever I can. So, yes! I will become a jolly guy. I'll do some man-about-town banter. Right ... NOW!

I spy a lady cleaning the outside of her house windows. She turns to smile at me. Here's my chance. Here I go. 'Keep scrubbing, ha ha!' I shout, in a friendly way. She flinches. Maybe it didn't sound friendly. I'm already *so, so sorry*. In case you missed that, I said, 'Keep scrubbing.' Keep. Scrubbing. I have my headphones in, so I'm not even sure if I said that, it might have come out as 'Keem Smubby!' or 'Beep Sluppy!' for all I know, I can't hear anything except George Harrison going on about the sun's imminent arrival.

The lady, in a nautical blue-and-white-striped long-sleeved T-shirt, keeps the smile frozen to her face but it definitely departs from her eyes, which now seem to be saying 'please don't talk to me again or I'll be forced to fetch the gun'. I hope to all the gods in heaven that I didn't just simply say 'scrubber'. Can't remember now. It's possible. Anything's possible. Oh my god ... this is dreadful. What a shambles. I'm not even past her yet, poor woman. It can't get any worse, at least. Unless. Yep, it can. I give her a thumbs up. Holy ... flip. I must never try to banter again. I should be legally ordered not to banter within a hundred yards of another human. Shamefully slithering my way back home, I skulk immediately to the living room, open my laptop and start looking for somewhere else to live. I hear Tuvalu is quite nice at this time of year.

17

I've always wanted to be a water guy. A sailor. With a beard. A boat fella. A chap who can fish, and teach other chaps to fish so they know how to fish. I hypothetically want to jump off locks in the summer until fishermen and barge owners and parents of paddling children ask me if I'd mind going away. Trouble is, I'm not really that into being wet. But as Britain is going through a heatwave, it'd be wise to be submerged in cool liquid right now, so long story short, I'm going wild swimming. I've also always wanted to experience the hottest day ever in the UK. I think I'll do that today, too. A BOGOF offer on adventures. It's the end of July and set to reach 39°C. That's hot enough to actually warrant using the phrase 'stay hydrated' instead of 'perhaps have some water now and then'. That's just about hot enough to turn an apple tree into a tarte tatin tree. So hot you could crack an egg on the pavement and, although it wouldn't necessarily cook, it would still get really quite warm. All the ducks on the river will be crispy by teatime. Granted, according to Google I've already experienced the UK's hottest day, in 2003, but that was at the end of my first year of uni, so I probably slept through most of it. Or watched the repeat of *Neighbours* with red eyes. We had a 'proper' summer last year, of course, but I can't really remember that either, apart from snatches of memories from the World Cup, watching a royal wedding on telly, fleeing from a garden centre but I still can't remember why – though I recall being there to buy a small ornamental owl to say thanks to Dad for sorting out my garden. Buying a ridiculously large beanbag. Never out of the same stained tartan shorts; always, always sweating.

I'm still suffering from the echoes of that time. I've just come out of hospital after a flare-up of pancreatitis. Shortly after the Blackpool and Spain jaunts, I was due to be best man at Chris G's wedding, and then go to the Isle of Wight to meet the team at Rapanui who make the *Very British Problems* T-shirts. Instead I was in Bay Tree Ward, again, doing shots of morphine, trying to ignore the spiders only I could see crawling over my blanket. I'm okay now, though still quite embarrassed about an incident in which I attempted to hand in a full, disposable wee bottle to a member of the public in the corridor (she was wearing the same blue as the nurses!). Now I have to take my car for its service and MOT.

'Good morning, Mr Temple.' Sean is the sturdy proprietor of United Motors in Huntingdon. He reminds me a bit of Dara Ó Briain but with a Geordie accent.

'Morning, how are you today, Sean?'

'Hot.' A loud machine does something to a blue hatchback outside.

'It's going to get even hotter,' says the customer in the vest behind me, sitting beneath a painting of pink flowers on one of four wooden dining chairs with green velvety padding, trying to control his chocolate Labrador. It's 9 a.m. and it's already 28°C and I'm in a jumper to hide all the holes in my arms. I've said the word 'hot' out loud at least fifty times. I'm acting even hotter than I feel, to be honest. It's a drama, being hot, as a Brit. You have to participate: you're a small but integral part of a large cast of downcast players. Every British person you currently meet is only saying 'it's so hot', 'it's too hot' or, like the man in the vest, 'it's going to get even hotter'. Brits are obsessed with it not only being hot . . . but it GOING to get EVEN HOTTER.

'Yes, thank you for that, sir, I know it's getting hotter. Thank you very much indeed for that. Okay, Mr Temple, that'll be ready, realistically, by late afternoon.'

If I could pick a way not to spend the hottest day ever, it's standing over running car engines. Thankfully I know absolutely nothing about cars, so if you did catch me doing that I'd urge you to call a doctor. Now I'm off to Wickes to buy some duct tape, or duck tape, or gaffer tape . . . certainly an important tape, given all its titles. The day has really started with a bang. My hay fever is in full bloom. Though it's not nearly as bad as it used to be. I used to have to stand in the shower breathing in cold water vapour just to open my throat enough for oxygen to get in. Looked like some horrible, twisted version of a Timotei advert.

The second my boring jobs are all done, it's time to give this hot day the cold solution it needs. I'm standing on the edge of a bit of the River Ouse on Portholme Meadow, England's largest water meadow (though the scale of its largeness changes depending on who you ask). I should be going through my publisher's first edit of *Very British Problems* Book

Four – it's only a few months until it's out in the shops for Christmas. My friend Adam ('B') and I will have to take our usual pilgrimage to the Waterstones in Piccadilly to buy one. The first time we did that, giggling at the till like naughty kids as we asked for 'a copy of the humour book *Very British Problems*, please, snigger', the assistant told us that although *Very British Problems* did make him laugh, 'you should check out *102 English Things To Do*, that one's really funny'. Next time we went we couldn't find *Very British Problems* Book Two, so we just went and had a Chipotle instead. But anyway, editing can wait: the river is calling me, like I imagine it calls trouts. Although trouts are already in it, so why would they need to be called? The heat is melting my brain.

I'd love to enjoy swimming. I've been meaning to try out the public swimming pool, but there'll definitely be people there, and I don't have the nerve for that today. Fear of embarrassment is a major reason for lots of people (I guess, I have no data) not doing stuff. B and I watched a clip on Twitter of a bunch of American news anchors dancing. The clip is titled, 'the whitest thing ever'. The dancing is like the sort of rap impressions your dad used to do despite you telling him not to.

'It'd be lovely to have such little sense of embarrassment, like those guys,' I put to B.

'Yeah,' he puts back to me. 'To live life knowing the truth – that nobody really gives a shit what you do.'

I'm reminded of my first-ever Very British Problems tweet: 'Walking back into the office after a slightly shorter haircut than normal'. The tweet of an anxious man. In reality, nobody notices your haircut. Especially if you're a bloke who's gone from short back and sides to ever-so-slightly-shorter back and sides. You just have, because of the way the chemicals in your brain flow, an inflated sense of your own importance in the world, but in an anti-confidence-giving way. They should change the name of anti-anxiety pills to 'realise nobody gives a shit about what you do' pills. Has a better ring to it than Sertraline. Of course anxiety is more complicated than just pure embarrassment, but that's certainly part of it. It must be so much fun not to be frightened.

I have a strong fear of being perceived to have done something in the wrong manner. Take the last stag do I attended, for instance, in Kraków, a stag do where we paid a dog to attack the groom (don't worry, Toby, I won't name you) and it ended up pulling him to the floor and humping his face. Anyway, in the apartment (scary room full of single beds) I was petrified of taking a shower. All the potential ways it could go wrong. I could use up all the water. Someone might come in. What if I break the nozzle? What if someone's waiting? I could slip and break my hip. What if there's nowhere to hang my towel? So, I don't have a shower. I watch everyone else go in one by one, come out clean, watch them spend an hour publicly getting ready, and I'm in awe. I'll be so worried about messing it up and drawing attention that I'll just not have a wash, and be the only person who looks an absolute state. Better to be dirty than risk making a mess of getting clean. Then I'll worry all day about looking dirty. I just could not go on these sorts of trips, but then that's wrong as well. Thankfully nearly everyone I know is married now.

If there's a plate of biscuits on a meeting room table, I won't reach for one. What if someone thinks I'm greedy? What if I pick someone else's favourite? I'll only feel stressed while eating it anyway. The crumbs! No, just go hungry and admire-while-hating the guy who picks up all the bourbons. I really do want to reach for a biscuit, though. I'm on the edge of a diving board, willing myself to pounce on the digestives; desperate to throw caution to the wind and say, 'Sod it! I'm having a Hobnob!' I also pretend to like and not like things, to fit in. Everyone does this to some degree, but I'll do it over the most trivial things. I remember at school, they used to do these burgers for lunch (back in the days when you'd just have an almost black burger patty on a plate, not your modern mid-rare bunned affair of today) which had cheese in the middle of the actual burger, all sealed in like an infection. Everyone absolutely despised them. To be fair, they did look quite gnarly. Trouble is, I loved them, so I used to pretend I thought they were just regular burgers, then I'd cut into one and go, 'Ah, disgusting, no, what have I done?' then only eat half of one while looking queasy. How I longed to eat the whole thing.

When I stopped working in an office altogether, it became far too easy to just stop living completely – no opinions, no debate, no grooming, no teeth-cleaning, no tastes, no inter-ests, no life – just a dead man shutting himself away, boxed up and stuffed in the wardrobe with his bowling ball and his golf club and his wrapping paper, and the bulging can of surströmming he ordered for an adventure that he can't bring himself to eat, waiting patiently for life to blow over. Month after month after month, trapped in a room, rotting like veg.

Fear of embarrassment from getting things wrong is why I don't go swimming, apart from the whole not-liking-being-soaked thing. I might muck it up. I'll look bad. I can't get fit because I'm, in my mind, too fat. The illogical ego of it. People will look at my belly and laugh. The one and only time I've used a public swimming pool as an adult was at Tooting Bec Lido. I had gout in my right ankle at the time, so I could only power myself on one side. I kept going in circles. Any great whites in the pool that day would've picked me off with ease. When I was out of the pool I was sucking in my body like I was trying to digest myself: all tensed up, red and square like Mr Strong.

I've been in the sea, of course, but I spend the whole time expecting to step on a living ball of spikes. The sea is too messy, too big, terribly damp. Worse things always happen there. I don't like being in it. I just like looking at it, as you know. I recently gave Stand-Up Paddle Boarding a go. It's a bit the In Thing. I don't want to talk about it. All I'll say is I managed to stand on the board for less time than you could stand a pencil up by itself. I was clattering about like a cup that doesn't fit the saucer. I spent most of the time kneeling, worrying I'd fall and drift out to sea like some shabby old shark. Of course, I only had one go, discovered I wasn't an expert yet, so that was the end of that. No, I'm not very good at balancing at all, although saying that, I did come within seconds of Chessington World of Adventures' bucking bronco record, but I was only a child so I hardly ever think about it at all. Literally seconds. If that old lady tripping over hadn't distracted me.

If I manage to stay out of the way of errant buses, I will reach my golden years and realise I've drastically overthought life. It plays on my mind. I'll get to heaven and I'll be sent back to earth for another go with the instruction: 'Once more with feeling.'

'You're brave!' says a lady in full hiking gear as she walks past me standing on the edge of the River Ouse in just navy trunks and a brand-new remarkably quickly acquired T-shirt sunburn, cold water up to my ankles. I'm not brave. I've been at this level of submersion for about fifteen minutes. Then, as if bungee jumping, I say 'sod it' and, rather than the dive I expected my body to do, scrape myself underwater like a croc.

I stay in there for about half an hour, only my head above water. Wallowing, hippo-like, watching barges drift by (terrifying from this vantage point, to be honest). I wish I had warpaint on my face. I feel faintly ridiculous, but mildly . . . free? If that's not too wanky? It's not like a bath, where I'm hot, faintly repulsed and waiting to get out (always been a shower man), and it's not artificial and trippy, like the flotation tank. There are no lanes or chlorine or timers. It's just refreshing. I'm sure you know what being in water is like, so not quite sure why I'm explaining so much; I guess it's just made me a bit giddy. Wild swimming (even though I'm not swimming, I'm just kind of bobbing) has been in the papers a lot recently, along with every activity ever. There must be something in it. I certainly feel refreshed as I clamber out, despite suspecting that I look a bit like I've escaped from a prison, albeit a prison where I've been well fed. Maybe I'll try a proper wild swim one day, in a loch or something, meet Nessy, get on the monster's back for a change, but for this afternoon, this little bit of river has been very pleasant to me. I walk back over the meadow (the UK's largest water meadow) like a low-budget Poldark, grateful for the experience, grateful to be healthy today and as zen as I'm capable of. Grateful to not be in a hot office. I wasn't even worrying about my phone getting wet, or sitting on the bank and being chewed up by a passing spaniel (not that I saw anyone daft enough to have their dog out in this heat), because I left it at home. It must be the longest period Twitter and I have been apart for nearly a decade. While 'my timeline' on Twitter was making jokes about the new prime minister and my Facebook feed was urging me to visit Blackpool Tower again, I was in a river. I was a crocodile. I win. My shoulders sting.

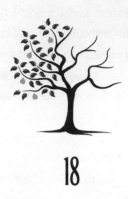

18

Digital detox, you say? Okay then, if you insist. Seeing as an hour or so without my phone made me happy, I'll do twenty-four hours. Although actually, I'm waiting for some important calls regarding various legal and medical things . . . so, let's make it twenty-four hours with no internet. No apps. No 'social'. Starting now. The Silicon Valley CEO types seem to call this one 'dopamine fasting' . . . taking away stimulants for a period of time, of which technology is predictably a big one – the freebase cocaine of geek buzzes – in order to feel a nice big fresh rush when you bring them back. Sounds kind of obvious, just like 'waking up earlier means you have time to do more stuff as long as you don't mind going to bed really early after a day of mostly showering'.

I must admit, I do feel a little proud when my phone tells me my screen time is down for the week, although saying that, for the amount I still look at it, it's a bit like being congratulated by a dietician for only having three pizzas in the night. Come to think of it, it's a little sinister, being congratulated by your phone for not looking at it, isn't it? A bit gaslight-y? Reminds me of a bottle of vodka telling you to drink it responsibly. 'Don't drink me – a dangerous, tasteless poison – in order to feel pissed, that's not the point of me! I'm your friend.'

I try to leave my phone alone as much as possible, but it's usually futile. I go on walks to clear my head but can't go more than four steps without lifting my Space Grey content crack pipe to my face. Take a hit, crave another, take a hit, crave another. Sometimes I pretend I'm looking at a map, scrunching up my expression in mock confusion and scanning the horizon, so other walkers won't think I'm just a screen junkie checking to see if I've bagged myself another 'like', as if anyone's taking the slightest bit of notice of me anyway. I do this in the supermarket, too: my 'I'm looking at my shopping list' mime, so the elderly people I'm constantly trying to impress won't suspect I've rudely just stopped by the chicken thighs to get a quick tweet fix. What a weird little world I've trapped myself in. Like any addiction, it revolves around paranoia, self-obsession, self loathing and chasing a forever dwindling satisfaction. I should attach my phone to a dumb-bell – I'd have arms like tree trunks. More likely it'd just live in the shed and I'd never go near it. Win-win.

Okay, digital detox, done that now. It was tense. I think an hour of digital downtime now and then should be fine. Any longer, and I really start to miss all the stuff on the internet. As I mentioned earlier, I try not to look at Twitter too much these days, despite my job being on it. I still look at it too much, though. I used to read books and articles. Now I mainly read reams of furious individual little opinions. If I overdo social media, I start to navigate towards people who seem to be obsessed with mental health, the people who spend all day tweeting 'remember to breathe', then I become obsessed with my own mental health in ways that involve doing everything but dealing with it.

I've even seen people on Twitter say they see their mental illness as both a superpower and, in separate tweets, like a broken arm (as in, mental health problems should be talked about and readily treated as you would a broken arm. Twitter is littered with crap, confused and largely unnecessary analogies about mental health). Well, how does that work? It's one or the other. Is your broken arm like a superpower too? Pretty crappy superpower. Is it a bird? Is it a plane? Oh, damn, no, it's Broken Arm Man, I guess we're all dead. A broken limb is a hindrance. If I had a busted leg, I'd want to try to diminish the bustedness as much as possible, even if the process was uncomfortable and sometimes painful, even if recovery encountered speed bumps and the leg never completely healed. I'd want it as 'better' as possible. I certainly wouldn't celebrate it, I'd work to rid myself of it. But saying all that is to pander to the analogy, one which just doesn't work. Broken limbs and mental illness – well, they're both health problems, but completely different ones. It's an analogy for analogy's sake; it's for retweets, and it's not helpful.

I also refuse to call it 'my anxiety', like it's a cheeky little pet. I see anxiety as primarily a medical problem, a chemical imbalance exacerbated by circumstance, situation and experience; it's a bloody pain, so I'll have some painkillers, please, doc. I went through a period when I thought it was some kind of rule that you *have* to talk about mental health on Twitter, that that was specifically what it was for. I started to talk. I even thought I was meant to become some kind of mental health guru and started posting tweets about kind-ness, sounding like a cross between a soppy birthday card and a horoscope. Then I'd sit back and wait for my reward: retweets. The more I talked, the more I began to see anxiety as a part of me; with relief I accepted it and settled for it. A big mistake. I broke through the stigma, then simply stopped there. This led to me being in a bedroom for years. I cultivated the illness, rather than attempting to diminish or handle it. 'No, I'm not going to try to leave the house today, I don't have to, I have anxiety, you see.' I don't want anxiety to be my personality. I don't want 'alcoholic' to be my identity. For me, the idea of 'if I have one, then all bets are off' excuses me of responsibility and seems like a self-fulfilling prophecy (though if the labelling system works for you and keeps you off the drink, then more power to you). If one must compare mental health problems to broken bones, then one (not sure why I've started talking like the Queen here) can't in the same breath treat them as special, or even valuable. 'Hello, I'm Rob, and I'm a broken arm guy' (round of applause). It's silly. Irresponsibly twee.

Too much Twitter and I drift off into a world of self-pity and introspection, which, to me, seems rather vulgar. 'It's okay to talk,' people say, which is a vital message for so many who get trapped in their own heads and think their world is helpless and hopeless and lonely, but you hardly ever hear, 'It's okay not to talk, too.' I started talking too much, online, to unqualified people, expecting magic to happen. I just sank even further down into anxiety quicksand. I'm not advocat-ing the stiff upper lip, or maybe I am, I don't know; maybe in moderation, if possible, if it works for you. Anyway, don't listen to me. I'm not an expert, not even on myself, let alone you. I'm just glad I can now identify the bits of social media that aren't good for me and try to avoid obsessing over them.

Well, got that off my chest. As Paul Merton might say on *Have I Got News for You* after a few minutes of discussing something VERY SERIOUS, 'That wasn't very funny, was it?' Now, if you'll excuse me, I have to catch up on what the Twitter strangers I hate have been bitching about in my absence.

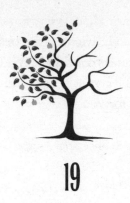

19

I love bees. You have to love bees. I have a T-shirt that asks, or rather tells people, to hurry up and save the goddamn bees. I like the way bees look – they're very stylish – and I like their work, specifically the manufacturing of honey. But if one comes anywhere near me I run a four-minute mile, zigzagging and flailing away towards the horizon as if dodging bullets. I imagine bees to be like mini killer whales. I LOVE killer whales, you have to love killer whales, but I don't want one thrashing about near me while I'm enjoying a salad.

My fear of bees stems, predictably, from being stung as a toddler. I've been stung many times since, once waking up at my sister's old flat in Finchley to find a wasp casually planting its bum in my thumb over and over again; once after sticking my hand over a wasp in my kitchen to stop Raffy slurping it up. But it was that first sting from the big fat bumblebee, who for reasons known only to itself wanted to end its life, that really got under my skin. That was the one that really stuck with/in me. Since then I've always thought I should make my peace with our friends, the bees. Also, I've seen what happens to Macaulay Culkin in *My Girl* – I don't want bees as my enemy. As for you, wasps, I'm sorry, but you can still sod off. No salad for you.

To: Cambridgeshire Beekeepers' Association
Hi there,
    I was wondering if I could talk to someone about possibly visiting you to be among bees? I love them, but I've always had a bit of a fear of them which I'd like to put an end to. And, of course, I'd love to raise awareness about how important bees are.
    All my best,
    Rob Temple

Susan
To: You
Hello Rob,
    Thank you for your email. Can you explain a little more about what you mean by 'being among bees'?
    Best wishes,
    Susan

Reading this reply, I can clearly see how my phrasing has made me sound like a danger. I send an email in return to assure Susan I'd simply like to put on all the protective clobber and have bees fly all around me. Hopefully this will make me sound less like I want to be some kind of god to the bees.

Stephen

To: You and Susan

Good morning Rob,

Your enquiry has been passed on to me as I am the manager [*my email has been escalated!*] of the CBKA Apiary at Wandlebury, not far from Addenbrooke's Hospital, which we use for the majority of our teaching.

I am happy for you to come to the apiary, and I will 'dress you up' and involve you in an inspection of the hive. It is of course dependent on the weather, but are you available during the week?

Regards,

Stephen

Result! What a lovely reply. I immediately feel this is going to be a rewarding and memorable adventure. We arrange for me to visit on the first Monday of August, with Stephen proposing we meet 'at the Bee Shed' at Wandlebury Country Park at 2 p.m. Wandlebury is about forty-five minutes' drive from here, just to the south east of Cambridge. I've never been, but it sounds like the kind of place that's filled with wild (not domesticated) berries, and jars of jam nestled in hay in little pine boxes; cloudy 9 per cent scrumpy and pubs with names like The Sparrow and Turnip overflowing with frothing ale called 'Wizard's Revenge', and other rosy-cheeked wholesome delights. Yes, that's Wandlebury. A magical place. I've basically decided, with no prior knowledge on which to base such an assumption, that Wandlebury is The Shire (anywhere in the UK that contains even the smallest patch of grass is liable to be called The Shire since the *Lord of the Rings* films came out).

'Excuse me, sorry to bother you, but do you know where . . . '

'STOP! Stop there, please! I'll come to you . . . wait!'

About five steps ago in Wandlebury Park, I stepped past a sign warning me not to pass beyond the point of said sign.

'Sorry, I'll go back!' I holler at the man in the dark green polo shirt (the ranger's favourite) who's bounding towards me over logs and long grass and bits of metal.

'No, no, it's fine, it's just there's a lot of dangerous machinery here, I don't want you to step on a rusty blade or anything.'

'Sorry, I saw the sign but I ignored it,' I say, not meaning to, which must sound quite ridiculous to him. Such a preposterous admission certainly sounds quite ridiculous to me as soon as it leaves my lips, but I'm in flustered mode now, so any old garbled nonsense will be about to throw itself out of my cerebrum. 'I'm sorry to bother you, anyway, honestly, but I was just wondering, I was wondering would it be okay if I just asked you a question, of sorts?'

'Go ahead.'

'Cheers . . . sorry, I don't suppose you happen to know where the Bee Shed is, do you?'

I've been sweatily stumbling around woodland for about forty minutes, a navy jacket zipped up to the Adam's apple, at one point accidentally venturing into someone's back garden, trying to find the elusive 2 p.m. meeting point. Stephen did attach a map to his emails, but in the car park I discovered it only expanded to the size of a postage stamp. I still have fifteen minutes until I'm officially late, but I'm flushed with panic.

'The Bee Shed?' the man replies, breaking into the smile people break into when they're about to tell you you're standing a metre from the Bee Shed. He points directly over my shoulder.

We share a chuckle over the close proximity of the Bee Shed ('What am I like!') as an estate car gently pulls up and parks. Out pops a slender man to rummage around in the boot. He reminds me a little of a slightly older Hugh Fearnley-Whittingstall. It must be Stephen, unless some madman has decided to go for a drive down a woodland path. Loitering near the shed, I unzip my jacket to reveal my bees T-shirt that's covered in bees (pictures of bumblebees, not actual bees); I feel a rush of adrenaline propel me to speak, like a firm hand from behind trying to push me into a swimming pool. Once sound leaves my mouth there'll be no turning back. Taking a few hesitant steps forward, a nervous man's run-up, I hope my brain has judged the volume needed to communicate effectively from twenty yards, and in my best 'Dr Livingstone, I presume?' voice, croak:

'Hi, is it ... Stephen?'

'Yes, hello, Rob?'

'Yes, haha! I'm here to see the bees!' I say, and then point to my T-shirt.

'They're the wrong sort of bees,' says Stephen.

I'd be quite happy to live in the Bee Shed. It has that same comforting, dusty, tumbling sunlight I so enjoyed in the antique shop in St Ives; they must order it from the same supplier. This wooden sanctuary is as relaxing as any flotation tank, reminding me of the 'summer house' (a shed with carpet) we had growing up. There's a delicious aroma, possibly imagined, of just-used lawnmower. They should make a grass-and-petrol scented candle. I'd like to sit in here every day of spring, summer and autumn until the end of my days, drinking nettle tea from a metal mug, wearing khaki waterproof trousers with a muddy multitool in my pocket, arms tanned and etched with bramble scratches, occasionally spurred into a fluster upon spotting what I believe to be a rare hornbill on a sycamore branch, or a curious ferret snuffling through the dandelions. Stephen and I could idly play Scrabble and chat about the predictions of frost.

The wooden floorboards bounce and creak; shelves neatly hang stacked with large metal tubs and containers, presumably for honey, reminiscent of the sheds of the most dedicated home brewers. Yes, this is the best shed I've ever been in (and I've been in some great sheds, believe me. I often go to the garden centre just to keep abreast of the latest ones, and also to have a fry-up). I'd be quite happy for this shed experience to be the entire adventure.

'So, why do you want to be a beekeeper?'

'I don't know if I do, really, but I'd like to find out if it's something for me. I'm a bit terrified of bees, to be honest.'

Stephen unlocks a cupboard and hands me a suit to try for size, as well as some wellies and long gloves.

'Just to be certain, this suit is bee-proof, isn't it, Stephen?' I half joke. Stephen pauses and begins his answer with, 'Well . . . ' Now ordinarily I'm sure this would worry me, but due to the woozy warmth of the shed and Stephen's calming manner, I take in the unexpected information that bee stings can indeed puncture the suit – say, for example, if a bee were to get crushed in the crevice of a bent limb, it might feel the need to lash out with the ferocity needed to puncture the suit and, in the process, your flesh – with uncharacteristic nonchalance (actual nonchalance, not the pretend stuff I usually deploy).

Suitably suited and booted, we leave the shed and stroll a short distance, looking like a nineteenth-century version of spacemen, making a sharp left over a low fence into a secluded bit of woods. Right there, just one step away from a public footpath, are hives containing thousands upon thousands of honeybees. 'They're really not altogether that interested in us,' Stephen assures me, as he marks down on a chart that, like most days, today the bees are at the maximum level of calm. You'd still get a fright if you jumped over the fence to retrieve a football, I think. The next hour or so passes very quickly. Stephen somehow spots a queen bee amid a pile of, to my eye, remarkably similar-looking bees, catches it in a little cage and marks it with a green pen, as I stand rigid as a beefeater, failing against my will to look chilled, while tiny fizzing asteroids bounce off my face guard.

'If you want to get away from the world, here's the place to do it,' Stephen continues, handing me a heavy shelf of bees, wax and honey. 'I pop down here for fifteen minutes and before I know it, two hours have gone by.' Maybe that's it: learn how to retreat from the world but in moderation. Not in a 'lock yourself in a room for ever' way. Maybe I'm concentrating too hard on how to be a participant in the world when I should be finding out how to find my healthy home from home away from it. Isn't that just what a hobby actually is? Is my sudden revelation literally just 'get a hobby'? Bloody hell, I think it is, you know. A GP once told me I'd benefit from getting a proper job, but sod that, so yeah ... I think I just need a hobby. One that isn't 'going to Blackpool'. It's possible I'm thinking too much again. I become aware that I'm staring into the distance again, face as blank as a mannequin's bits. I should be concentrating on the bees. Wow, there's an awful lot of bees.

I'm pretty sure I won't recall many titbits of information

that Stephen's feeding me, not for the want of trying but due to my Pavlovian jumpiness and terrible memory (and it's hard to type iPhone notes with oven mitts on), but I do know I'm having a lovely time just listening and occasionally saying, 'Oh right, I see.' It's hypnotic. I feel grateful to be here CHRIST THERE'S A BEE ON MY HEAVILY PROTECTED HAND! ARGH!

Before I know what's happened, we're back in the shed. I ask the question I've been saving up. 'Stephen, can I just ask, does local honey really cure hay fever?' Immediately I get the sense that Stephen must be asked this a lot, a theory backed up by him telling me that he is asked this a lot (you're much better off with tablets, is the gist of the answer). He's already locked my suit away in the cupboard when I realise I've left my phone in one of its pockets. We're exiting the shed and I wonder, should I just abandon my phone? Doing so might be ... good? Don't want to cause a fuss. No, I should say something, and I do, and it's no trouble. I climb into my car, somewhat drained but also buzzing, remove the 'Attending Beekeeping Meeting' sign I was told to put on the windscreen to avoid parking fees (I wonder if that sign could work just about anywhere? Would it be powerful enough to frighten off London traffic wardens? 'Hey, man, don't mess with me, I'm a beekeeper!'), and I follow Stephen to his house. Don't worry, he invited me to do so. I purchase two pots of Cambridgeshire honey, one runny and one set. He only sells to those in the know, you see. For the first time in my life, legally at least, I'm a preferred client. When I arrive home, me, Mum and Dad have honey on fresh white bread with cups of tea, and we talk of how kind Stephen was to show me the bees and how tasty the honey is.

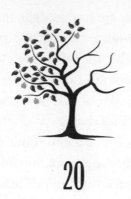

20

'You know those barges that go up and down the river?'

'Who?' I'm thinking about bees, not paying attention.

'The boats, you know, on the river?' repeats Mum from behind her iPad.

'Oh. Yeah?'

'Did you know they have toilets that just empty straight into the river?'

'Really?'

'Apparently. That's what you're swimming in. Mess.'

'Is that true? I'm sure that's not true.'

'I just read it on Facebook.'

'Great. I might go back to thinking about bees now.'

'Good idea.'

Surely the boat bogs don't just empty into the river? That doesn't sound right at all. Otherwise what's to stop people from just going in an old plaster of Paris bucket and sloshing it over the side? Or just cutting out the middleman (the bucket): some sou'westered fiend hitching down their waders and dropping a brown anchor straight into the drink? My desire for blissful ignorance trumps my quest for the truth, and I avoid googling the matter for my own health, instead looking up why the heck it's called plaster of Paris ('Known since ancient times, plaster of Paris is so called because of its preparation from the abundant gypsum found near Paris' – britannica.com). Then I go back to thinking about the bees. I enjoyed Bee Day. My experience of being among the bees with Stephen has reignited my love of being taught. I spend a lot of time worrying that people hate me, but with teachers I can make sure I come across well; I can be attentive and polite, feel the satisfying glow of being the best student.

I did well academically because I didn't want to let the teachers down. Bosses have always been pleased with me (which is like the diet version of being liked), and it takes exceptional circumstances for me to miss a deadline. I love haircuts and doctor's appointments, because I'm not in charge, I'm the passive participant in the game. I dislike being the expert. This is why I like being medically examined. I find it quite relaxing (maybe this is why I keep making myself ill); as long as there's no pain, all you have to do is sit and absorb. When I was little I pretended to have a broken leg; I wouldn't quit the act until a doctor had pretended to fix it. As an adult I don't even have to actually learn; I can be super-passive and relaxed about the absorbing knowledge part of things. There's no exam. Sometimes this does mean I'm concentrating more on being conscientious than on what I'm being told (I'm heavily reliant on the post-meeting follow-up email), but as long as the teacher doesn't know I'm just acting at absorbing, I can't see the harm. I also make sure to remind myself that often the expert, like me, must be simply trying to get through the day, so as long as I'm polite and nod at the right places, everyone's happy.

With this in mind, and encouraged by the success of my bee adventure (nothing went badly wrong), I decide to book a tour of the Tate Modern with an art historian. People always wish they could sing or draw. People who can't do those things, I mean. Is it possible to be good at singing and drawing at the same time? Must be. Actually, yes, of course it is. David Bowie could do both. Bob Dylan. John and Yoko. Anyway, given the choice, I think I'd choose drawing, because if I could sing I'd be too shy to show off about it. I'm not saying drawing is all art's about, but it seems to be a key part to a lot of it. You can probably tell I don't know much about art, other than I like staring at some of it. I need to know more about art, yes yes.

I pull into St Pancras (on a train, I'm not just propelling myself along like some sort of speedy eel) at just before noon on a steamy mid-August day. The Pink Line snakes its way east with me in its belly – sitting with my case between my knees, near to where two carriages join, the rubber attachment bellowing in and out like an accordion – all the way to Whitechapel. The wheels on my case rumble and roll over uneven paving, and are frequently yanked up over holes, saliva, gum and kerbs, for half a mile to a lockbox on a lamp post on Dunbridge Street. It's nearly time to check in to an Airbnb. Not *quite*, though, so I walk back to the Underground station and do the walk again, a mistake on such a warm day. Peter, my host, is in the hallway of the stylish modern flat, walls adorned with what I soon learn are his own artworks and photography.

'Hey, how's it going?'

'Really good, thanks, do you mind if I come in? Sorry, I didn't mean to just let myself in, it's just you said to use the lockbox, I didn't want to ...'

'Come in, come in, can I get you a cup of tea?'

The railway seems to go right under the flat. There's a little bag of foam earplugs in my room for bedtime, though I'm used to and enjoy train noise, having had the ones to Victoria zooming by metres from my bedroom window when I lived with Tori at 11 Byrne Road.

I have a bad back, and the skin's peeling off my hands, some of the physical symptoms of anxiety that I enjoy, and I'm sweating like the duck and hoisin wrap I'll soon discover in my rucksack, a side effect of my recently upped medication, which is also currently making me feel pilled-up, my brain fizzing out of my scalp and through my hair like an aspirin. The side effect warnings that come with meds make me think of a Peter Cook quote: 'Now I tell you the downside of this is you feel awful, but the upside is you feel terrific'. It doesn't help my perspiration problem that it's also bloody hot. Peter is a photographer, with long hair, tats and what a man who buys his clothes from Tesco (Hi) would describe as 'rock star clothing'. He has a sideline in selling leather bags sourced from Morocco. Maybe I should try to haggle for one using my mad bartering skillz. The back of my head is a waterfall of sweat as we drink our tea and chat about marketing, and I'm very aware of how moist I am.

Sweating isn't too bad, though, in the grand scheme; it's a shame that it's an effect of both the condition and the medicine – double sweat! – but you can always towel off. The physical symptom I first encountered at the start of my experiences with anxiety was shaking. It blighted my life; couldn't do anything in public. Now it's reasonably controlled through medication. It manifested when I had to give the first presentation of my life in sixth form, which broke my brain. 'Look, even his head's shaking,' someone said as I vibrated my way through a short talk. It was in a psychology lesson (cruel irony). As Dan H finished his section, he handed control of the overhead projector to me and my hands started shaking, magnified in huge shadows on the pull-down screen as I tried to manoeuvre my slides. It looked like I was doing a puppet show of two turkeys having a seizure.

In an attempt to control the hand situation, I gripped them tightly to my legs, sending the shivers upwards. I'd simply shifted the nervous energy to my head. If only it'd been a physics lesson, I could have cracked out an awesome Isaac Newton joke, thereby causing so much hysterical laughter and rolling around that the attention would have been directed away from my wobbly skull. I looked like David Gray singing 'Babylon', only in silence. At that moment I knew I would never have the confidence to present the Royal Variety Performance. I'd never be Speaker of the House of Commons.

So as not to impose, I've vacated and left Peter to the comfort of his flat. I've been wandering around Shoreditch for hours, stopping to have a good stare at various places ... the Cereal Killer Cafe, a ukulele shop, a menu in the window of Dirty Bones. When I get back at 10 p.m., there's no sign of Peter, and lovely aromatic smells are coming from the kitchen. It's crowded with young Japanese women, all gathered around the oven, seemingly finding the task of cooking absolutely hilarious. Scents of chilli and ginger make my mouth water as much as my neck. My dinner, to be taken when safely locked in my room, is a packet of Roast Beef Monster Munch.

When to go to the bathroom? The sun has risen again, the trains are in full chug, and I've spent the last few hours listening for a sign that it's safe to prevent my bladder from exploding. And that sign finally arrives in the form of rustling and stomping and zipping, shortly followed by that of the front door closing . . . followed thereafter by beautiful silence.

My quick showering (they could return at any time!) has made me sweat even more. Like the old towel riddle goes, the more vigorously I dry, the wetter I get. I'm not built for summer. It's about an hour's walk to the Southbank. Even though I wasn't born in London, and I only lived here during my twenties, I still consider myself a Londoner rather than a tourist. It's like being in the army: once you've lived here you always have the badge of honour. This means I stride in London, like a Londoner, with speed and purpose, always with the sense that I know exactly where I'm going. I didn't spend a decade learning the tube map off by heart to be mistaken for an amateur day tripper down here to look at waxworks of William and Harry, thank you very much. Arriving at the Tate in what seems like mere seconds since I left the flat, I realise I can't remember a single bit of the journey; it's like I've sleepwalked here. I often have these autopilot blackouts when I'm nervous.

Julia's sitting at an al fresco table at the Terrace Bar on level one of the Blavatnik Building. She's wearing large shades beneath a sharp fringe. Why is everyone so much more fashionable than I am? With my shorts sitting just above my pale knees, rugged mountain footwear and trusty green backpack full of emergency things, I look like I'm doing my Duke of Edinburgh Awards.

Julia did her MA in History of Art Photography in London and began training on the Tate Volunteer Guides programme, starting to deliver free tours shortly afterwards. 'Then I had a stint as an assistant researcher at Tate's collection research department, which gave me an interesting insight into how the gallery's labels and online texts are written,' she tells me as we stroll through the lobby, both trying to match each other's pace, which always results in a slow walk. 'I wrote my thesis about one of Tate's exhibition displays, so basically I was spending all my time here, either researching, explaining contemporary art to the visitors or looking around. After my graduation, I decided to combine all of my passions together and came up with the idea of the Art Walks. I love art, walking, researching and storytelling – that's how the idea of NEJA's Art Walks was born.'

'What does NEJA mean?'

'NEJA is my creative nickname, my photography alter ego, if you like, but I thought it could also stand for "New Electrifying Journeys through Art".'

I like that. I need a creative nickname. Something like . . . 'Man Ambles Around Aimlessly'. People could shout it at me as I amble past. 'MAAA!' they'd bleat. 'MAAA!'

Now I must confess, else I won't sleep, that I've tried to dupe you. It's true that we strolled slowly through the lobby, but everything you've just read about how Julia got into art tours, she actually told me, on request, via email after the event. I was too nervy and discombobulated to ask about her background at the time. Plus, and this is rare for me, I didn't have a pen.

'So, Rob, do you have any particular art that you like?' Julia really does ask, live in the Tate, in an Eastern European accent, which she tells me is a mixture of Lithuanian and Russian, 'A bit modified because I've lived in the UK for so long.'

'Not really,' I reply, in my Mr Bean accent. 'Erm . . . I guess I've always liked Van Gogh?' I say this with a tone of slight embarrassment, like I've just told a top chef that my favourite meal is toast. I mean, yeah, toast is genius, everyone likes toast, but it's a bit obvious.

'Did you hear about this?' Julia asks, as we pass a sign inside the Tate telling us the tenth-floor viewing platform is closed. A couple of days ago, a teenager picked up a little six-year-old French boy and dropped him off the side of it. He fell 100 feet to the fifth-floor roof. The news report kept mentioning the sound of the mother's screams. Somehow he survived, but is in a critical condition.

'I did hear, absolutely terrible,' I reply as we enter the packed lift. As we stop off at floors on the way to ours, people get in and out and Julia and I are obliged to do-si-do our way around the metal box, me whispering 'sorry' on repeat. I see Duchamp's urinal, and a colourful installation based on Brick Lane; Roy Lichtenstein's *Whaam!* and other groovy bits of art. At one point we're told to *ssh* by a security guard. No talking about art, please, this isn't the place! My back keeps twingeing, which means I spend most of the time walking around at a 90-degree angle. Still, it's nice and cool inside and Julia is a pleasure to listen to. 'When we've finished the tour I'll give you the number of a good acupuncturist . . . for your back,' she says, and she does. We say goodbye on the Southbank and I spend the rest of the day trying to get lost.

The next day, as I'm preparing to depart the Airbnb, dead on the 11 a.m. checkout, I notice that Peter has a unicycle.

Horrible flashback. I lived with a girl who started going out with a professional clown, I was told, after we broke up. This suspicion was confirmed one night when I was helping her load some things into her car and spotted a unicycle in the boot. 'Have you seen any really long shoes by the door? Found a red nose in the bathroom lately?' Big Dan asked when I told him about the unicycle, which was very funny.

Looking back at my art adventure, I had a nice time. I'm aware that I most fully enjoy things in retrospect, but I'm also learning, through therapy, that this is okay, and what everyone does, to varying degrees. It's not some personal affliction. You can only complete an experience once you've viewed it with hindsight anyway. And that's okay, even if, yes, I'd prefer a bit more 'loving it in the moment' moments. Relief-fuelled reminiscence is good enough for the time being. Better than not enjoying things at any time at all. The relief after the event is my reward for getting out and doing something. Taking myself on adventures is like taking slow-release opioids – still worth it even if Elysium takes a while to reach.

I've just read it's part of what's termed 'deferred gratification'. Damn, I thought I'd made it up.

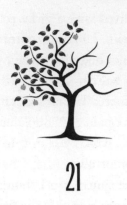

21

Beekeeping, or bee observing, followed by walking around looking at art, makes me keen to keep this adventure momentum rolling. Back in Godmanchester I book a hot-air balloon ride to lift off from Ferry Meadows (*not* England's largest water meadow) in Peterborough. I grew up just down the road, spending weekends cycling around Ferry Meadows with Mark. It would be lovely to go back. More and more this year I'm realising how much I enjoy being up in the air looking down on land. Perhaps it's a result of Big Dan's *Lord of the Rings* role playing by the lake – it's stayed with me as a symbol of the value of getting out and seeing panoramic vistas, being able to sweep over them, from the right vantage point, with one thick brushstroke of your hand. My mind obviously wishes for me to seek these moments, again and again, because it knows they make me happy. How's that for a fancy way of saying 'do what you like'? The flight requires setting off tomorrow down the A1(M) at 4 a.m. for a sunrise flight with a dozen or so other people; all couples, no doubt.

It's getting towards 11 p.m., so I ring the pilot as instructed to check we're still on for lift-off in the morning. 'Due to strong winds, the flight will not be going ahead, please rebook …' Of *course* the weather's too awful for a hot-air balloon flight, it's the middle of summer in Britain! What did I expect? My first feeling is relief. I've paid to not do an experience: money well spent. Hopefully I'll have dreamt up an exciting alternative adventure by tomorrow.

I wake in bed, at the time when I should be coming in to land after an hour of floating around the sky with strangers in a basket. It's for the best I didn't have to rise at 4 a.m.; I was knackered last night and needed to get straight to sleep after ringing the pilot's recorded flight update hotline, so naturally I picked up my phone again and before I knew it, I could hear birds singing while I wearily read about the manufacturing process of Branston Pickle.

Teeth-cleaning means staring at your own face for a good two minutes. Unless you're one of those people who clean their teeth while walking around a kitchen breakfast bar going through your mail, like in the movies ('Honey, what's this letter?' It's always either really bad/good/exciting/dramatic/life-changing/shenanigan-inducing news, and the character with the toothbrush can somehow tell this purely by the plain white envelope). Bathrooms should have tellies as standard. God, I have a stupid face. It's a bit more crumpled than yesterday, and the day before that. Not too shabby, mind. Luckily I have a secret weapon, my trusty Boots No7 'Protect & Perfect' moisturiser, which helps to stop my skin having the texture of an ultra-durable Bag for Life. Mum makes Dad use it now, 'else he gets a bit leathery'. The good thing about two minutes of teeth-brushing, aside from protecting your enamel, is that it leads to fanciful ideas. Have you ever noticed how many ideas you have when staring idly at your own face? Maybe it's just me. After ten seconds of puzzlement about why I'm consistently older rather than younger, I start to think about what I can do to not waste the day. There must be another adventure to be had. Perhaps it's something about the shape of my toothbrush, but I suddenly remember how Mark has often talked about seeing some crocodiles at a nearby farm. I loved the bees, so yes ... I should be among the crocodiles. That sounds like a nice little adventure.

Maybe that's it ... animals should be my life. It's been staring me in the face. I even started my career at *Your Dog Magazine*. I recently found all the old issues in a box in the garage behind my weights bench, and flicked to one of my features at random. 'How big is Britain's dog poo problem? Rob Temple reports'. Next to this in big letters: 'SPEAK OUT! Is where you live spoilt by dog poo? Send your letters to Rob Temple, *Your Dog Magazine*, Roebuck House, 33 Broad Street, Stamford, Lincolnshire'. I never looked forward to my post arriving. 'Oh no, Sheila from Loughborough has found another turd in her garden.' I was so nervous at that job, straight out of uni at twenty-one, in a small, friendly publishing house in Stamford next to my school. I remember the terror of having to talk in editorial meetings. And having to prepare five mugs of tea and coffee every two hours and then, like Julie Walters with two soups, rattle them into the room. The mugs shook so much on the flimsy metal tray, it sounded like I was coming down the hall, past the *Your Cat Magazine* and *Horse & Pony* offices, firing a machine gun.

You find the crocodiles at Johnsons of Old Hurst Farm a fifteen-minute drive away. They have three Nile crocodiles,

Cuddles, Sherbet and Romeo. It's high time we all met. It's the school holidays, so I'll set off for opening time, beat the rush.

'I'm off to see some crocodiles,' I sing to my parents to the tune of 'We're Off To See The Wizard'. They're enjoying tea and toast in the kitchen, sunlight from the pleasant, not-windy-at-all day thickly rollered over half the table. They both sit on the same side like newsreaders, facing the telly, so when entering the kitchen you can pretend you're walking into an audition or job interview.

'Crocodiles?!' Mum blurts as her white china cup connects with her saucer with a delicate clink.

'Yes, at that farm Mark goes to down the road.'

'Well, I hope they don't ever come here.'

'Come here?'

'If it floods, they could get in that river and end up floating down here.'

'I don't think they're ... loose? And the river's miles away, they're not going to climb out of the river and walk down the road to the house.'

'You never know, Robert,' she says knowingly.

'What? You think three crocodiles might come to the front door and ring the bell, disguised as delivery men from Amazon?'

'You can't rule it out.'

Dad looks at me with an expression that says, 'Your mother's got a point.'

Mum, who, by the way, has seen *Bridget Jones's Diary* at least fifty times and has an obsession with Queen and the Queen, has a way of stating her case that leaves you somewhat bewildered yet also unable to argue against it. She also has a habit of stating that she's not very smart, which is patently wrong, as Dad is always quick to counter. They're a fine team. Dad, who likes puzzles, sums, owls, gardening, typing with his index fingers and the Sunday papers, is a highly organised man, obsessively so, and is deeply set in his routines. He recently said, 'It upsets my dishwasher routine,' about me using a plate at an irregular time. He once took me to the McDonald's when I was little, but wore a suit and ordered the sophisticated option – the Filet-O-Fish – in case he happened to bump into a client. He sometimes says, 'I just go with the flow,' but that's only if he knows exactly to where the flow is going. He has a total of thirteen clocks in his study: on mobiles, house phones, two plastic weather station things and two regular wall-mounted clocks. There's even a third clock on a wooden pencil holder. I'm not going to count that as a standalone clock. That's a combo clock. Dad is so often seen fiddling with clocks that my niece, Freya, when asked, 'What do you think Grandad did for a living?' answered, 'Clock-winder?' He's a gentleman, a pretend misery, he can't abide bullies, always tells us how early he wakes up and that he'd worry if he didn't have anything to worry about. Mum and Dad would truly be incomplete without each other. Mum digs out his reluctant silly side, which would otherwise remain buried deeper than the dinosaurs. She's worried his memory will start to slow one day, but there's no sign of that yet.

'Okay, I'll see you later.'

'Will you be back for lunch?' asks Dad, reindeer mug lowered to half mast.

'Should think so.'

'Hmm.'

Pulling into the gravel car park, I'm crestfallen to see it's absolutely rammed. The whole of Huntingdonshire woke up this morning and decided to meet crocodiles. They must have a good PR team. This is too many cars. People are reaching dead ends and panicking, violently reversing and jerking around, ten-point-turning all over the place, like fifty goldfish in a tank built for two. I nearly rolled my car traversing a pile of gravel, but have luckily managed to safely deposit it half in a bush.

For some reason I'm rushing, half jogging past the farm shop and tea room, past a donkey and some meerkats, up the ramp, dodging between toddlers and prams into the platform of the steamy Tropical House. There they are: crocodiles. I look at them for all of five seconds, take a photograph, jog back to the car and drive home, feeling annoyed with myself. This adventure was really just a box-ticking exercise. Deep down – well, not that deep down, really, in fact quite shallow down – I knew I wasn't really fussed about seeing crocodiles, as spoilt as that sounds. I don't want to see them by myself. It's the kind of thing, for me anyway, that requires someone with whom to go, 'Ooh, look, crocodiles!' If you say 'ooh, look, crocodiles' out loud to yourself, people back away. Trust me, they do. I should've dragged James along. It's like sightseeing by yourself. How long do you make yourself look at a really tall building before thinking, 'Yep, that's a building,' and moving on to a really old bridge? 'Well, it's no great disaster, get over it,' I tell myself, which I quickly do. It's just that sometimes I don't feel like I'm really here.

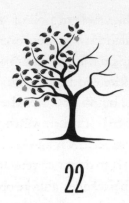

22

I tried to see the world, and I managed a few days in one street in Barcelona. Now I have the chance to see the world all in one go, thanks to an artwork called *Gaia*, a floating 3D replica of Planet Earth, by Luke Jerram. It's in Peterborough, at the cathedral, so I can make up for my failed hot-air balloon visit by journeying there to see what's essentially another big balloon. There's something poetic about seeing the whole of the planet from my city of birth, I think. The installation is smaller than the actual earth, I imagine so it would fit: 1.8 million times smaller. By my calculations I make that 'around the world in eighty steps'. It rotates once every four minutes, 360 times faster than the friendly rock it's based on. Its message is to inspire us not to ruin our only home.

I'm getting all this from a feature on the local news, BBC *Look East*, which we're watching (which we always watch) after tea (curry tonight, penne tomorrow). My parents love the local news. They love all news. They mainly sit through it to get to the weather report. They trust the telly weather above all else. They treat it like the exit poll of weather. The apps, the hearsay, the internet, the numerous weather stations, the ACTUAL OUTSIDE … According to my parents, all of these might very well give you a rough indication of what the weather is/will be like, but if you want the ultimate meteorological tip-off, you need the telly weather. Though saying that, once they've seen the telly weather, even then do they almost immediately start to doubt its veracity, so they wait for the next one. Like with packages, they're obsessed with when weather is 'meant to be' arriving. Even if it has little impact on their plans. 'It's meant to be windy tomorrow,' Mum'll warn, as if it means it'll be windy in the lounge and we must batten down all the decorative stags and vast collection of remote controls in preparation for the strong easterly breeze of 2019. 'It's cold in here,' they'll say, when it's 24 degrees. They'll also say, 'It's hot in here,' when it's 24 degrees. It's always 24 degrees. Mum constantly wants the fire on, as well as the heating, but Dad puts up a resistance as he doesn't want to use up all the logs.

'I might go and see that tomorrow.'

'Ooh, that's a good idea, you could park in Queensgate,' suggests Mum.

'What's he on about?' Dad asks. Since I've been back living here he seems to ask this after most things I say.

'I might go to Peterborough Cathedral to see that big earth, Dad.'

'Oh, sounds like a good idea to me. I wouldn't mind seeing that myself.'

'Do you want to come?'

'No.'

'Okay. I'll go in the morning then, after breakfast.'

'It's a huge building. You've been there before, haven't you? It costs a lot to upkeep.'

The next day, still a little puzzled as to whether Dad thinks I'm going to Peterborough to refurbish the cathedral, I have a breakfast of various things eaten while standing in the cold glow of the open fridge. I really must stop eating like this. I wouldn't be surprised if I add 1,000 calories or more over the recommended daily intake with this habit. A forkful of pickle here, a sly slice of Stilton there, a gentle tearing of ham, a deftly plucked tomato from the ever-half-full Spode salad bowl on the bottom shelf. I have measured out my life with coffee spoons of half-inched coleslaw. I regularly have to use the handheld Dyson to give the bit of floor in front of the fridge a quick going-over. It's an uncouth habit, fridge eating. After I clean my freshly stained shirt with a wet wipe, I drive to Peterborough. The clock on my dashboard reads 12:34 – the time that follows me around. Rarely a day goes by when my eyes are not on a clock at 12:34. The phenomenon of synchronicity, says Google. As an accountant, my dad's personal time stalker is more complicated than mine: when he looks at a clock, which is often, the numbers usually add up to a five or a seven.

Parking on level seven of one of the four multistorey car parks (2,300 spaces in total), I take the stairs down to level five – 'TO THE SHOPS [*downwards arrow*]' – and march through Queensgate shopping centre, the main hub of the city, and of my life, really. It was born in 1982, a year before me, and, unlike me, was opened by Queen Beatrix of the Netherlands. It has a massive John Lewis. Chris G and I would meet here as teenagers, in that frustrating age just before you can get served in pubs, back when the height of cool for a teenager was to own a Storm watch, and spend our Saturdays marching around aimlessly. I've known Chris since I was eight. Since we got mobile phones at around fifteen, there's been hardly a day that we haven't talked to each other, usually about nonsense. We used to watch episodes of *Who Wants to Be a Millionaire* over corded landline phones. I like daft people, especially ones who you really have to prise the daft from; when you're one of the few allowed into the silliness inside their otherwise serious heads. 'A little nonsense now and then is relished by the wisest men', as Mr Wonka said. Chris is a legal and political expert and lives with Shirin in Woolwich, and is my dear friend with whom I share a large set of our own personal customised memes. If you and a companion don't possess the same or similar chemical equation of daft – not that you even have to show it, but it has to be IN both of you – then you've as much chance of interesting each other as do a cod and a cow.

Past the massive John Lewis, soon followed by the clothes and homewares bit of M&S, past Next and down the escalator, past the food bit of M&S and a right at the big Boots, past Clintons, and you end up at the end of Queensgate that has the place which makes the giant cookie cakes opposite McDonald's – which as Chris first observed makes it the sweetest-smelling 'just outside McDonald's' area ever. This particular McDonald's has a layout which makes it always look too busy. To the side of it are the doors which take you out or in from the market square, on the corner of which you'll find the archway through to the cathedral. This is where my earliest memory was filmed: little me inside a buggy, my roof a transparent cover dotted with raindrops, Mum's face blurred above it, extremely comfortable and safe. 'You used to make me pull that over you even if it wasn't raining, to stop all the old ladies saying hello and pinching your cheeks.' It'd be nice to think I've matured a bit since then.

Walking through the manicured lawns dotted with cross-legged, sleeves-rolled-up lunch break folks munching tuna baguettes and superfood salads, open bags of salt and vinegar crisps and popcorn and pretzels propped up in the grass below the statues of St Peter, St Paul and St Andrew, who reside on the three high gables of the cathedral's West Front, I walk through the large doors to go from warm August sunshine to fusty tomb-like cool. It smells like an AA meeting. There it is, the big little earth, two hundred metres away, behind a huge hanging Christ on a crucifix, about twenty people gathered around it. I wonder if God is looking at it too, thinking, 'I made that! Took me under a week! Then I retired. Bosh!' It's really quite impressive. Larger than it looked on *Look East*.

I feel a bit of a plum trying to take a photo so it looks as if I'm holding the thing, but I've had 'I've got the whole world in my hand would make a great Instagram caption!' in my head since last night, so there's no turning back. Everyone's taking photographs from all angles, so everyone feels they're in the way; there's a lot of polite ducking going on, even though the exhibit is hanging high from the cathedral roof. I really like this big little earth, and I don't feel alone here, looking at it; there's a sense of community and camaraderie as we all gather round the globe. Maybe it's because we're in a circle, which is the only way to huddle around a sphere. Or we're all just digging the chilled churchy vibes. Maybe we're all facing how fleeting our time is together, the message of the piece hard at work. Maybe everyone's actually really miserable; I don't know. I wonder if there's a 1.8 million times smaller version of me somewhere on that earth, fretting about my recent haircut and a million other miniature worries. I'm feeling kind of wise, like a monk. Might put on some brown robes and walk slowly.

'Mummy, what's it made of?' says a little boy dressed as Batman.

'I don't know, darling, what do you think?'

'Is it plastic?'

'Wouldn't that be ironic?' I think to myself and smirk, like a dickhead.

'It might be, darling. It looks like a balloon, doesn't it?'

'It's full of poo!'

'Thomas, shush, please.'

'It's full of poo-poo!'

Overhearing the poo conversation has snapped me from my reverie, ruined my philosophising, killed my zen. It's thrown me, is what it's done, and causes me to stare into space for some time. When I come to I'm aware that I'm glaring, with my resting cross face, at an elderly gentleman in a motorised wheelchair, who's glaring back at me. Must say something. 'Impressive, isn't it?' I shout towards him. I haven't used my voice for over an hour, the volume's out of whack. He rides away.

I put some change in the collection box by the door – gotta keep the Big Man happy – but nobody sees (apart from Him) which disappointingly makes me feel a bit disappointed. There's a flatscreen TV showing a quote from way before Jesus was born: 'If you do not change direction, you may end up where you are heading'. A good driving tip; I'll keep it in mind on the journey home.

Nipping into M&S, I pick up parmesan, tikka-flavoured

chicken pieces and some other fancy bits before getting in my car, excited to upload my photos to social media. As mobile phones have become smarter it takes me longer and longer to actually start the car. I'll be typing and uploading and liking, getting my fix, for at least half an hour before I finally release the handbrake and trundle off.

'So, how was it?' asks Mum, crunching on her Lotus biscuit in the lounge.

'Yeah, not bad, good, really great. Just like on the telly, really.'

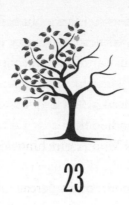

23

At the age of thirty-five, I really should be capable of growing a proper beard and chopping down a tree. I'm acutely aware that, although there's no shame in it, I'm living with my parents, living quite a silly, childish life, compared to, say, a fireman, or a surgeon. I mean, look at House, he was meant to be my age in the first series of, well, *House*, and he was Head of Diagnostics at a major hospital. I'm buying celery jars for larks and writing about it. I need an axe and facial hair. A nice thick beard for winter. Not a hipster beard. No. I have no interest in craft beer or neck tattoos of swallows, or beard oil; no desire to be a cheeky waiter in a meat restaurant who sits on a turned-around chair to take your order with the pen he keeps behind his ear. I want a big, wild, scraggly beard; to be the wild man of the Fens. I've given it a lot of half-arsed attempts since my chin started whiskering, usually persevering for a couple of weeks before I concede that I look like I've hit hard times and fire up the BaByliss i-Stubble clippers (0.4 mm setting).

During my teens I was so in awe of my hairier chums that I even experimented with a chestnutty-coloured Just For Men on my patchy goatee and mutton chops. The hair was so whispery the dye went straight through and stained my face. My sideburns looked drawn on, like I was some kind of Lego butcher, while my mouth looked as if I'd recently attacked a chocolate cake sans cutlery. A girl I fancied said, 'Aah, look at your little beard.' Yeah. If my parents threw the classic 'If your friends jumped off a cliff, would you follow them?' at me, I'd think, 'If those friends had beards and the leap resulted in thicker face foliage for me, then I'd be off the side of the rock face before you could say, "Stop it, Robert, for god's sake".' I've had a crack at cultivating thick fuzz biannually since the Just For Men debacle. Friends, partners and family have, universally, said to me, 'You look much, much better when you've had a shave'. I refuse to listen. I start to grow a beard and they look sad, or concerned, or they simply laugh and say, 'Looking a bit woolly, there.' Thank you, I reply.

The skin underneath my facial hair – hair which can't commit to a colour scheme, so goes with a jazzy mix of red, grey, black, orange and white – turns dry, scaly, sore and spotty (weren't they Bash Street Kids?) but still I push/grow slowly on in anger – the beard version of slamming a slow-shutting door. I haven't shaved for three days now, and up close I'm starting to look like a non-bald Phil Mitchell after a week on the Bell's, as is usual at this stage. I've dressed in my most lumberjack shirt and I'm off to the shed to fetch the axe.

Wow. Axes are heavy. The one I'm holding feels as weighty as a whole salmon. A fat one, at that. I've helped myself to this axe from Dad's shed. Mum's warned me I'll never be able to chop the logs she's arranged for me to have a go at, that they've gone too hard since they stopped being part of a tree earlier in the year. We'll see about that. I'm feeling strong. I'm a bull.

'This shouldn't be a problem, Mum.'

'Don't hurt yourself.'

'Stand back!'

Pulling the axe up and hoisting it over my head and so far back that my belly pops out to say 'Greetings!' from under my vest, I take a breath and bring the chopper down, light speed, with all my worldly might. The axe is nothing more than a blur and I thrash it towards its target. *THWACK!* Vibrations rattle through my triceps. All my energy has been transferred from my core to that of my enemy: the log. The log remains whole, almost completely unblemished. I fear I've broken my spine. A few more attempts should do it. THWACK! THWACK! *THHHHHWACK!* Catch my breath. Thwack. One more go. Tap. 'Shall we go back inside now?' Mum asks. 'Okay, I think ... I think ... [*breathe*] this ... this log must be ... faulty.' Stupid log. Stupid axe!

My face is itching like crazy as my sweat drips into my whiskers, so I replace the axe, enter the house and razz the whole sorry palaver into the sink. Adventure over. Trust me to try to grow up in the most basic, childish and literal, visual way possible. I blame my school and their forced use of briefcases.

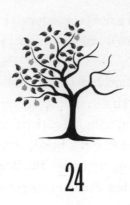

24

Music festivals were everything to me, in my salad days. My 'falafel and salad in a pita bread for £8' days. Four days mashed in a field was my idea of a real swell time; the ultimate summer holiday. But with each passing year my enjoyment gradually cranked down in correlation to my packing notching up. I started off by queuing for entrance with a spare size small T-shirt, a toothbrush, a multipack of Frazzles and a dazed look on my face and ended up, years later, with enough gear – the practical type of gear that you get from Millets, not the herbal kind – to survive a polar expedition. An assortment of plasters, emergency flare and spare pillowcases? Imodium and Dioralyte? Literally preparing for the imagined inevitability of soiling myself? Not very rock 'n' roll. The moment you start to worry about getting mud on any one of the five pairs of hiking boots you've packed – that's when you know to give up on Glasto. But darn it, yes, I said darn it, I don't want to give up, I want to get back in the game. There's only one man who can help me now.

Chris (also known as Woody, along with a raft of other names) is my festival right-hand man. Festival tales are as boring as the retelling of dreams, but I can say that we had some good times, once including infiltrating backstage (okay, just one tale) by authoritatively and urgently, as if we were on a life-or-death mission, telling security that the folded towels we were holding were 'for the band'. Towels for the band, you say? Right this way, sir! I hear The Beatles stopped touring because staff at Shea Stadium forgot to provide enough fluffy flannels.

Chris is one of the best of them. We met in school and were happy being silent together, surely the mark of true friendship. He's also a crazy man. A maverick. He was an usher at my wedding, but he might not have made it because he'd 'left a motorbike in South America and might have to pick it up'. He's a marvel, nobody knows what he's planning. And parents love him. Anyway, he's cycling down from London (only sixty-odd miles) for the weekend and we've decided to buy tickets at the gate for the We Out Here Festival's inaugural year. It's a jazz festival on the grounds that used to host the Secret Garden Party in Abbots Ripton only a ten-minute drive away. We attended the first one of those. And the second. Slept with our heads in a puddle of red wine; long, pink, crispy hair for three days. I'm not sure if we knew just how much fun we were having. I suppose you don't when you're having it. I'm not really into jazz, but I imagine it'll be quite a small, relaxed affair with decent toilets, like those you get at weddings: they still smell of blue chemicals and sewerage, but are painted racing green and have a jar of plastic flowers between the two sinks and Vivaldi piped in from somewhere as you tipsily style your hair for the twenty-fifth time that day and nervously say, 'How's it going?' to the father of the bride washing his hands next to you who you've not yet said hello to (and you're the groom!).

Chris arrives, and click, I am comfortable in my skin again. My dislocated personality has been popped back in. I revert to a relaxed, confident, happy me, and I'm relieved to know that me still exists. I know when I'm with close friends because we don't shake hands and my hands don't shake. This is one of the frustrating things about anxiety: your mind resists giving the green light to things you know will be good. I try to put off seeing my friends as much as I can, even though it's without exception always a delight.

'Oi oi, how's it going, me old grape?'

'Good, thanks, mate, how was the cycle?'

'Bit of a bloody nightmare to be honest, mate. Janet, how's it going? Great to see you ... Paul, how you keeping? Been well?' A big hug each for/from my mum and dad. I give Chris a glass of water and an apple – 'mate, I'd honestly say this is probably the nicest apple I've ever had' – before we take an early-evening walk to Portholme Meadow (the world's largest water meadow). Sitting on the tatty wooden bench by the lock, facing the expansive green baize stretching, dough-like, to Brampton, we chat for an hour or two about all the things we need to chat about, yearning for the past while ignoring the future, as one by one the sky pots its colours: blue, pink, black.

'I'm thinking, right, how nice would it be to be like those guys I was telling you about at the chilli festival?' I put to Chris while holding a fully loaded shard of poppadom, which breaks and sends shreds of raw onion and gloopy mango chutney all over Planet Spice's freshly laundered tablecloth. There was only so long we could sit on a dark meadow eating wine gums and rose-tinting on and on about the days of greasy hair and acne. Planet Spice, with its bright yellow and red decor, a scheme favoured by icons such as the Cozy Coupe children's car and McDonald's, Christ I think about McDonald's a lot, is much warmer than a field.

'How do you mean?'

'I dunno, like, being so into one particular thing. Being obsessed with chilli, so that's all you enjoy talking about, you know? Having a passion. Must be mega-nice to have that kind of focus. Mega into chilli! Surely it makes interacting easier? You've got your chilli mates, and you talk about chilli. You know where you are. You know?'

'I dunno, mate, I much prefer having a conversation with people who are into all sorts of stuff. If you got mega into chilli, I dunno, all we'd talk about is chilli. Also those guys aren't probably just into chilli, it's just that day you were at a chilli festival.'

'Yeah, you're right.' I realise I've been patronising the chilli people.

'Okay, I have one chicken madras ...'

'Thank you.'

'One mushroom rice ...'

'Cheers.'

'Vegetable sagwala ... and one garlic naan. Can I get you anything else to drink?'

'Nah, that's great, thanks, lovely, cheers very much.'

'This looks ace. But yeah, they say you've got to find what you love,' I continue, while touching the hotplate to confirm it's as hot as I've been warned.

'Yeah, but if someone's only into chilli, it isn't a bad thing, it's just . . . you're into loads of stuff, you can't force yourself to just pick one. I dunno, mate, just seems unnecessary.'

'Yeah, I guess so. Shall we get another rice?'

The next day it's pissing it down. The weather reporter on the telly warned, 'Unless you have to go out, it's best to stay in,' which is really my philosophy whatever the weather.

'They'll be having a miserable time at that festival,' Chris says in the warmth of my parents' living room.

'Yeah . . . listening to jazz soaking wet in the cold.'

'Sloshing in the mud to a snare solo? Luuurvely!'

'Maybe we could go later on if the rain stops.'

'Yeah, let's see how we feel. What shall we do now then, champ?'

TripAdvisor, what have you got for us in the local area? Something suited to a couple of likely lads with starry eyes and a to-hell-with-it attitude.

'We could go to the Oliver Cromwell museum in Huntingdon?'

On the mile walk to Huntingdon, armed with brollies, we stop in the sprawling Cambs Lock Antiques to rifle through unloved vinyl and blow dust off sherry glasses. These places really make you desire tat. Maybe I need to buy this broken accordion? Maybe I need another celery jar? Arriving at the Cromwell Museum in a building that used to be his and Samuel Pepys' school, next door to Pizza Express where they probably went at lunch break, we're greeted by two gentlemen who together, over an hour, provide us with everything you'd ever want to know about Cromwell but were afraid to ask. I do my usual thing of letting the imparted knowledge wash over me like sloshes of warm bath, while Chris actually engages, fires out question after question. For me it's a lecture, for him it's a seminar. He actually seems to know an awful lot about Cromwell, which he never mentioned before, though I appreciate it's not the sort of personal info you crack out at a party. I feel like I'm back at school. I feel the urge to lark about. It's a feeling I'd like to bottle.

'Large chips, curry sauce, Diet Coke and a tea, please.'

'No tea,' the man serving us at Barney's Plaice tells Chris.

'No tea?'

'No, we don't sell tea, sorry, only cold drinks.'

'Ah, okay, no worries.'

We sit in the window opposite St Mary's Church – next to Steve's Taxis and *The Hunts Post*, the view through the glass warped by drizzle, horses racing on the little telly in the corner – and rain salt and malt vinegar down into every nook and cranny of the styrofoam tray between us. We chat about Cromwell. A plaque on the wall a few doors down says the poet William Cowper used to live here, quite a while ago. He's the bloke who first said, 'Variety is the spice of life'. Spice! He must have been talking about Barney's curry sauce. He also coined 'God moves in mysterious ways', but I can't think how to link that to chips. I struggle to recall a more perfect weekend, from the best-ever apple to the best-ever meals in the best company. Thank goodness for rain. We decide to sack off the festival, before the owner of Barney's arrives to place in front of us a freshly brewed cup of tea. Praise the lord.

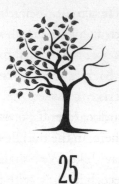

25

Why am I not cycling ridiculous distances? Eh? You tell me that! I know how to ride a bike. I own a bike! And a really hefty lock that was pretty expensive. I should go on a big long cycle ride, somewhere idyllic and warm, and find someone else to pay for it. I could say it's for climate change.

I roll Bakewell, my cherry-red Peugeot 206 that I've had since I was eighteen, back a bit from the garage door; I keep Bakewell at the marital home to both protect all the crap in the garage and to make burglars think someone still lives here. Sliding the grubby metal white door up, tearing a load of old cobwebs in the process, I'm faced with piles of boxes full of the stuff I lug from one home to the next, as well as empty boxes that once contained new appliances. I'm not sure why we all imagine that one day we'll fancy boxing up our microwaves and toasters in their original packaging, but you need Kondo levels of discipline to just bin them.

There's an old Domino's pizza box with half a pizza still in it ... when did I eat a pizza in the garage? Should I ...

take a bite? Hmmm. Better not. There's not one but three pop-up tents, a lot of tents for a man who now thinks camping is wank, and a neon-green battery-powered lawnmower with wheels caked in dry mud. The floor is covered in rusty leaves the texture of crispy seaweed but not nearly as tasty, and random bits of cardboard and polystyrene. It's all a bit haunted house. And there, in the middle of it all, lying on its side, is my black and navy bike. We bought two of these, both the same, for £199 apiece, but Rhi's, with the added luminous mudguards and bag rack, was stolen from the station on one of the days I wasn't fit to drive her there. I pop into the house to check for Tupperware boxes in the kitchen cupboards to later take back to my parents' house (my cupboards are 50 per cent reusable water bottles, 30 per cent Tupperware and 20 per cent half-full tubs of smoked paprika and empty soy sauce bottles) – they'll come in handy when we really start motoring with cooking all the apples.

I'm cycling to St Ives (again, the Cambridgeshire one) on a test run, before I commit to crossing Ecuador for the climate. I think my bike needs oil or grease or something, I don't know, I'm not a . . . bike mechanic? but it's quite stiff and hard to pedal. I'm hoping it'll loosen up as I go. To get to St Ives requires crossing the park, freewheeling down Silver Street, cutting through New Street and St Anne's Lane, hanging a right on Cambridge Road, past the White Hart and one of the Co-ops, under the bridge that until a clean-up recently was always caked in pigeon mess, out of Godmanchester and down Cow Lane. At the bottom of Cow Lane, past the sewage works, sits the Godmanchester Nature Reserve, where Raffy loved to run. He'd pelt it down the muddy tracks as if he was in the Grand National; he was about the size of a horse, as well. You turn right before the nature reserve and cross the field of cows to The Hemingfords. It's all going smoothly so far, just like riding a bike, ha ha. I should've playlisted some happier music for this adventure, though. Last time I saw a gang of cows, on Portholme Meadow (the solar system's largest water meadow), I was happily listening to the sweet harmonies of The Beach Boys. It made the cows look blissed out and peaceful. I remember thinking, 'Look at those lovely cows.' Today I'm listening to The Chemical Brothers, which is making the cows seem sinister. They look like they're scheming against me. I'm sure they're not; probably just thinking about grass. Aside from the menacing cows I'm feeling pretty at ease in general, almost to the point of experimenting with gear changes, as I power past the big houses on Common Lane. Within half an hour since I left my garage, I'm passing the Axe & Compass, which has a big playground in the garden that James loves. In the summer it serves barbecued burgers and coleslaw, or 'slaw' – chosen from brown-paper menus with no pound signs – in cute cardboard boxes.

It's just started spotting with rain. Not to worry, I'm wearing a waterproof jacket. I churn on, a bit tired now, heading out of Hemingford Abbots towards Hemingford Grey, home of The Cock, a fine country pub, great in winter, which plays audio from *Blackadder Goes Forth* in the toilets. There's a fire, ales, roast dinners with giant Yorkshires, sticky toffee puddings, fresh fish options on blackboards and people in waxed jackets and wellies. It's quite posh, in other words. I'd love to stop in for a bowl of fancy pork scratchings, especially as it's raining a bit harder now. I push on. Getting a bit chilly now. It's very quiet. The sky's quickly developing a dark contusion, swelling like a bicep that's been whacked with a steel bar, and the temperature drops another notch. Eerie. It feels like there's a flooded canopy above me, about to be poked with a sharp stick. Oh, hell. It's been poked. Biblical rain. Bloody hell. Hair wax stinging my eyes. My waterproof jacket has decided it's simply a regular jacket. Someone somewhere must be building an ark, because this is ridiculous. I'm turning back. It's a lark, getting caught in a downpour with a mate, running to shelter in a fit of laughter, shouting out at the absurdity of it all. Getting caught in one by yourself is just wet.

CRACK

I nearly fall off the back of the bike passing The Cock. Ouch. There's something remarkably wrong with my saddle. I stop to slick my hair back, rub my eyelids and see what we have here. What we have here is a completely broken saddle. It comes off in my hand. As I said, I'm not a bike mechanic by any stretch, but I know that for a saddle to be functioning at optimum level it should not be completely detached from the bike frame and being held in a hand. Christ's sake. Some sort of nut, or bolt, or some bit of important metal seems to have decided it's had enough. I have five miles to cycle, holding a saddle, soaking wet, standing enough so that an exposed rusty metal pole doesn't go up my arse. A Land Rover drives by and sprays me with mud.

Onwards!

My thighs have turned to hot stone. I've no choice but to walk my bike back in the downpour. The cows, sheltering together under green and purple trees like huge bunches of grapes, look at me in silence. They think I'm an idiot. My headphones aren't working any more. My jacket is clinging to me like wet tissue. It's turned into an umbrella-rammed-in-a-bin kind of day. I'm in the flat fenland of Cambridgeshire, a few miles from home, in daylight, and I'm pretty sure I'm close to death. It's a damn good job I'm not in Ecuador.

Shutting the garage door on my bike and its saddle, locking it in with the pizza again, I squelch back to Mum and Dad's, as moist as a good lemon drizzle cake.

'You're all wet,' Mum informs me.

'Yep.'

'Did you get caught in that rain?'

'Think so.'

'What on earth did you go out in the rain for?'

'It wasn't raining when I set off.'

'Yes, but it rained while you were out.'

'I know.'

'Chucked it down! Dear me. Don't you sit on any of the sofas. Go and have a shower.'

'Okay.'

'Put your clothes in the washing machine first.'

'Really?'

'Yes, come on.'

Dad walks in from the living room with a tray holding one empty reindeer mug and one empty china cup and saucer. I'm standing by the utility room in my pants. Nobody should ever be this naked in their parents' kitchen at thirty-five years of age. 'Still raining out there, is it?' I go up the stairs on all fours because my thighs have stopped working. The absolute state of me.

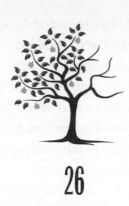

26

When you were little and you'd blow out the candles on your cake, what did you wish for? I understand if you don't want to say. Well, I used to wish for a chocolate factory. Sometimes I'd also wish for this crazy neon slide park I'd designed to be hidden through a door in the back of my wardrobe – in fact, I still wish for that sometimes – but I knew that was being a bit greedy. I think I just wanted to make my wardrobe a happier place, seeing as on the front of the door my parents had hung by the neck a life-size clown. It used to kick me when I'd walk past in the night to visit the bathroom. Sometimes I still see it. Its eyes, black crosses, as dead as death itself. What? Oh, yes, the chocolate factory. I always wanted one. Back then I simply didn't consider the logistics of running a successful confectionery business, I just fantasised about lakes of chocolate and everlasting gobstoppers.

Today I am going to make that fantasy a real adventure. No, I'm not going to buy a factory, I'm going to visit Cadbury World in Birmingham. At least, I was. That was the plan up until a few days ago, before my cavalier crunching of a mint imperial. Instead of being on my way to choc town, I'm at the dentist. Halfway through eating the mint, I began to think, 'Hmm … this mint is getting crunchier the more I crunch it.' Spitting it out, I went on to discover just how tricky it is to separate a ball of mulched-up mint and shattered tooth shards into their component parts. The two substances look remarkably similar.

The dentist is in Buckden, a village about five miles away. Catherine of Aragon, buried in Peterborough Cathedral, was confined here – not that that in any way helps you to picture the place, but it might come in handy in a pub quiz. I've left myself a lot of time to drive there, through puddles and over all the toytown bridges of two villages in The Offords, and the rail crossing which likes to stop you for at least fifteen minutes per visit.

'Hello, I have an appointment for … Temple?' I notice there's no bowl of mint imperials on the reception desk.

'Lovely, have a seat!'

'Cheers, thanks.'

I sit down in a chair with my back to reception and pretend to read a newsletter article about molars, while a woman opposite pretends to talk to her toddler. She's really talking to everyone else in the waiting room in code, saying, 'I'm a good parent and I'm trying my best to stop Samuel darling from ripping up this book'.

'Do you watch rugby? My husband's obsessed with it,' the receptionist says.

'No, I'm not really into it,' I reply, turning round to see that she's obviously asking her fellow receptionist, who has since come out of the back office to join her. Perhaps I could take off one of my shoes and crawl into it? Mortifying, but expected. Of course, this is nothing compared to my worst waiting room experience. I'd walked out of the GP surgery to find my car blocked in in the car park; one of those car parks that's a perfect square with one entrance/exit, designed for forcing polite confrontations. 'Excuse me, sorry, erm, does anyone in here drive a Renault Laguna? No?' All eyes in the (full) waiting room locked on me. Silence. Everyone gawping, like curious horses – in my memory they're all slowly chewing – as if I'd just marched in and said, 'Excuse me, would anyone care to dance?' You'll have gathered by now that I'm quite easily embarrassed, but having to loudly say the word 'Laguna' to a packed room . . . My god.

As I wait for the redness in my cheeks to die down, a woman in a large wide-brimmed hat that wouldn't look out of place at a wedding comes down the corridor to book in a follow-up appointment.

'Certainly, would you like a morning appointment or . . .'

'Afternoon would be better . . .'

The hat woman and the receptionist both laugh raucously. Louder than I've ever laughed in my time on earth.

'If possible!'

Both continue laughing. I'm worried they might laugh their heads right off.

'Three thirty?'

'Great. Actually I'd better check with my husband first, if that's okay!' More laughter. Almost belly laughter.

'That appointment would be with Lauriana.'

At this point, a posh elderly man in a waxed jacket, waiting with his wife, pipes up to contribute, 'Lauriana? Sounds like an HGV convention.' Wow. Astonishing. What a simultaneously quick yet bizarre joke. Everyone's laughing now. I wish I'd never eaten that bloody mint.

'Mr Temple?'

'That's me!'

The dentist takes me away to the drilling room. She'd seen me for an emergency appointment immediately after #mintgate, just to assess the damage; now she has the task of repairing the tooth. Aside from having to avoid eye contact with someone two inches from my face, I'm quite relaxed about the whole thing. All I have to do is lie here, and seeing as I'll have a mouth full of tools I won't have to make any small talk. None that makes sense, anyhow.

'What music would you like to listen to?' asks the nurse. I've never been asked this at a medical appointment before.

'I don't mind,' I reply, obviously.

'ALEXA ... PLAY ... COLD ... PLAY,' she shouts over her shoulder.

It's an odd experience, having two people in face masks looming over you, tinkering around in your mouth to the sound of suction, both singing along to 'Fix You' while they literally fix you.

'Nearly there, how are you doing? All okay?'

'UH-HURRH.'

'Not in any pain at all?'

'ER ... HAUUGH ... UH.'

'Good.'

The dentist asks me to check if my tooth feels even. It doesn't. I say I'm not sure. Maybe, I add. 'You don't sound sure.' She does more work and asks me to check again. Yes, that's better, that'll do. 'But is it perfect?' Yes, good enough. She does a bit more to it. 'How about now?' I hope it's okay, as again I move my tongue towards it. I feel like it has to be okay now, like I've run out of self-imposed attempts to adjust the amount of cheese I want at the delicatessen. It's perfect! And it actually is. Thank god. Lovely. Off with the yellow glasses and onwards to reception with numb lips to give them all my money.

The level crossing makes me and a conga of cars wait for twenty-two minutes on the way home. Looks like rain. Sky's hanging as heavy as a blanket of fag smoke on the ceilings of The Royal Oak where I grew up. Trains hurtle back and forth to London. Mouth still numb, my face as dexterous as bum cheeks. I'm not meant to eat for a few hours, but I have a bag of Skittles in the cupholder and who could resist? I'm writing my next *Telegraph* column in my head. It's on Very British Problems with owning an exotic pet. Up go the gates, five minutes till home.

'Hi.'

'How did you get on?'

'All good. No problems, all fixed.'

'Oh, that's good.'

'I'll be back in a sec, Mum, I've just got to go and write my column.'

'What's it on this week?'

'Exotic pets.'

'Ooh, that's a good one,' Mum says. She says this whatever the subject of the column.

'Yeah. So things like spiders, snakes, iguanas ... you know? Anyway, won't take too long ...'

'Armadillos!' Mum shouts as I walk out of the kitchen.

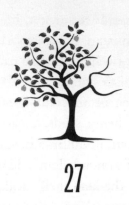

27

It's Monday morning and me, Lisa and Pete have driven to the Costco in Stevenage in their Skoda Yeti. 'Pete needs to come so I don't lose control of my spending,' Lisa says. I've recently embarked on a bit of a plan-cancelling spree. Some of those plans I feel it was wise to scrap, particularly the ones based in pubs, while others I annulled simply because I couldn't be arsed to de-arse myself from the sofa. I'm acutely aware of how quickly I could slip back into complete isolation. It only takes a few steps backwards to get stuck in a bedroom again: very easy to re-enter, very tricky to exit, in my experience.

So this adventure is purely about rebooting myself; jumping back, or forward, into a 'yes!' frame of mind. And I think if I can say 'yes!' to driving to a warehouse in Stevenage on a damp Monday, I can say 'yes!' to just about anything. It's nice to see Lisa and Pete as well; it would've taken some freakish amount of willpower to travel to a giant metal shed full of stuff I don't need on my own.

Before we set off from Lisa's house, she shows me just one of the many, many things you can buy at Costco – a place I've not visited before – a chunky tub of collagen. Apparently it's something to do with the keto diet. It lives on the 'keto shelf' in Lisa's kitchen in Stotfold. The shelf, in the cupboard, also contains hemp seeds, cacao powder, coconut flakes and coconut flour, psyllium husks, maca powder, raw cacao nibs, blanched almond flour and spirulina powder. The kids' shelf below the keto shelf speaks more my sort of language: Lucky Charms, Weetos and a large chocolate egg. Funnily enough I was reading about Weetos just the other day, on one of my 1 a.m. Wikipedia safaris, taking particular interest in this trivial titbit: 'The original mascot, introduced in 1987, was a skateboarder named Derek, who "*found life really boring, until new Weetos came out of the blue!*" delivered in a broad West Midlands accent.' Being so bored that you get excited about cereal … been there, Derek, my friend. Lisa makes me a cup of tea with milk and sugar. Well, not sugar, but something which looks exactly like sugar, called '100% Natural Erythritol'. Sounds about as natural as polystyrene to me, but that's an assumption based on no knowledge of the product whatsoever. Pete arrives home from doing some personal training work with a client and we set off, cutting through the clear blue day along the A1 southbound.

Turns out I like everything about Costco. It takes my breath away, like when I first saw Las Vegas. The sheer scale of the place dizzies me (in a good way). It really does appear to sell everything. There's more gear in here than in Del Boy's flat. It reminds me of when I'd go to the cash and carry with Dad as a teenager and we'd return home victorious with a whole box of Walkers crisps, a crate of apple Tango and a sweet shop jar of cola cubes . . . made me feel like a pharaoh.

One of the first things I see in this palace, this 'Costco', is a £35,000 engagement ring, which is kind of a double-edged sword when you think about it. On the one hand (where the ring will live), your fiancée will probably be quite chuffed with such an expensive sparkler, whereas on the other hand, explaining that you bought it in a Costco rather than, say, Tiffany's, well, it might take the shine off the gesture.

Pete and I wander off with one of the supersized trolleys that make everyone look like Borrowers, past a mountain of Superdry jumpers towering over a designer dining table that's next to a mini snowmobile, towards a giant red sign that says PIES, ROTISSERIE CHICKEN, BEEF, losing Lisa in the process (not intentionally, as if she were some kind of cop and we were looters on the lam, not like that. Our pockets are swag-free and Lisa's just a normal citizen visiting Costco for reasonably priced sushi and a mixed sandwich platter).

'Hang on, I'll call her,' I tell Pete, just as she appears from behind a tower of crystal decanters.

'Sorry,' she chuckles, 'I got stuck talking to the collagen lady.'

So much food. A whole salmon! £20! I don't know if that's good for a whole salmon, but . . . it's a whole salmon! 'Look! Chopped liver! Pete . . . Lisa . . . look . . . Pete . . . Pete . . . Lisa . . . look . . . what am I? Chopped liver?!' To help you paint the picture, I'm saying this while pointing at a number of tubs of chopped liver. I don't think they hear me properly because they don't laugh very loudly at all, but before I've had time to dwell on it I'm gently squeezing a vacuum pack of octopus tentacles like it's a fishy stress ball. This place is like Toys R Us for adults – it's brilliant, the wonders are thus far refusing to cease. It carries the same fascination as 'supermarket abroad on holiday'.

'Look at all those strawberries!'

'The size of that Lurpak!'

'Golf clubs!'

'Prawns!'

'Basketballs!'

'Tyres!'

'Pineapple chunks!'

'Fizzy laces!'

'Deckchairs!'

'Olives!'

'Tellies!'

'Dry shampoo!'

'Eggs! SO MANY EGGS!'

As Pete observes, there's something about Costco that forces you to walk around just saying what you see, like a basic version of the TV game show *Catchphrase*. You can even buy mayo in a big white plastic bucket, again the type of bucket you get plaster of Paris in . . . the type of container Gordon Ramsay finds in a nightmare kitchen's broken walk-in fridge, opening it up to the shock of a dripping pork joint looking as if something's just given birth to it. Four and a bit years past its 'best before' date and highly likely to contain plague, Chef Ramsay will quickly deduce that it's no good for eating and will declare that it could very easily 'BLOODY KILL SOMEONE! I'M CLOSING DOWN THE RESTAURANT! SHUT IT DOWN! LOOK AT THIS THING! LOOOK' [*Gordon takes a bite of it*] 'DISGUSTING! LOOK AT IT! I'VE EATEN THIS! I'VE EATEN IT!!!'

I don't need anything in here, but I want it all. I want to point at it all, to pick it up (and drop it and smash it into pieces, as is the case with the metre-long chocolate bar that slipped through my butterfingers), to say 'Wow! Look!' about it. I could live here. I should live here. I should buy these gloves, they're just like the pair I already own, but cheaper! I should buy this box of nappies in case I find a baby! I should buy this kettlebell – the ultimate toe-stubbing device! In the end I restrain myself and only buy the essentials: a vat of flying saucers (you know, the sweets that taste like chewing an envelope containing a speck of sherbet) and a pillow-sized sack of Indonesian crackers.

I'm glad I came (I really am, just in case this has all read like I've just discovered the thrill of sarcasm and wanted to have a really big go at it). And I'll come again soon, if only to try the beef hot dog and soda (with refills) for £1.50. If it provides anything like the pleasure I derive from tucking into IKEA's meatballs, then I'm in for quite the ride. OMG, they even do rental cars! They've got an optician's!

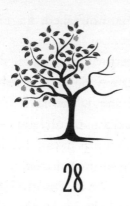

28

I've been somewhat obsessed with the idea of moving back to London. I feel as if everything since I left at the end of my twenties has been a blip, and that my returning to the capital will right the blip. It probably sounds like I'm trying to go back in time, which I know from experience and textbooks is notoriously tricky, but I've no desire to be the guy I was. I've learned lessons; I'm trying to be a better person. I was typically self-obsessed when on the sauce. You have to be. A lot of work, expense and time goes into such carefully maintained and measured self-harm. You hope to keep hold of your partner primarily so you have your own nurse. As you sink you drag them down with you. You lose them, your senses, and everything else that you love and need is lined up for the losing. A doctor will tell you what you need to do to cure yourself – stop ingesting the poison, numbnuts – and despite being the one who's booked the appointment, you'll say, 'Nah, there must be another way.' I'm still pretty self-obsessed, *he wrote in his memoir*, now that I'm trying to keep dry, just not as useless, unwashed, ungrateful, self-pitying and nasty with it.

Twice this year I've put down rental deposits on shared places, one in Highgate and one in Finsbury Park, only to back out at the last minute, which has been costly. I panicked to the point of physical and mental paralysis as the moving dates loomed closer. But I'm trying to build my confidence back slowly. After my successful trips to Peter's flat and to the Tate with Julia, I decide to bite off a bit more in the hope that it's chewable, and have booked a four-night stay close to Finsbury Park station. I found a flat, owned by Tina, an academic and writer who teaches yoga at Glastonbury each year, and thought it looked a suitably sensible and relaxing environment. It's the zenith of summer, and I'm about to set off. I have no other adventures planned, but there'll be no shortage of them to find in the big smoke, I'm sure. It's very hot.

Godmanchester was uncomfortably toasty when I set off this morning, but the late-August lunchtime London sun is a different beast entirely. It's positively villainous. The entire heat of the cosmos is currently concentrated over Haringey. There's a small child somewhere in space burning us all like ants with his giant magnifying glass. It's the type of weather that wants you dead. The air seems to be coming from a hairdryer. There's no choice but to sweat. CHRIST, I'M TURNING INTO A PUDDLE OF LIQUID SKIN, MELTING LIKE RED LEICESTER IN A TOASTER. Did I mention it's hot? I lollop slowly under Stroud Green Road bridge, against the flow of people heading towards the station, past the rows of vacant tents and empty sleeping bags, soundtracked by a man blowing a groggy blues through a golden saxophone. The melody is drunken and slow, like the last record player on earth on its final few spins.

Continuing past the hand car wash – please, spray me! Turn your jet washers on me, for I melt and spoil like cream! – I wind through a few streets off the main drag and locate Tina's building. By this point I've rubbed my face and neck raw with the hand towel I'm holding because the sweat keeps coming. Trying to keep myself dry is counterproductive, but I can't not try. Tina isn't in. Relief. I can sort myself out before introduction. Lockbox. Stairs. Fiddly lock. I'm in. A quick scan of the areas of the flat I'll be using: the bathroom (very central in the flat and no window, argh) and the bedroom (neat, modern, comfy, view of flats, windows only open a fraction, hot). I told Tina I'd mostly be out and about, being an intrepid adventurer, so I start as I mean to go on and search online for shenanigans.

So far, my adventures seem to be leading me to two things: water and food. It must be confirmation, a sign, that deep down I want to be a fisherman. Or a sea cucumber. Today it's water. It must be the heat. All I want to do is jump in the Thames. Years ago, for their anniversary, I gave my parents a couple of tickets for a meal on the Thames (on a boat). They often mention it as one of their favourite days. I think about doing it myself, but quickly disregard the notion. Silly idea. A solo romantic meal on a boat while a live band plays 'Fly Me To The Moon' would probably end with me jumping overboard weighted down with a rucksack full of cutlery. I need something a bit more thrilling. 'Speedboat through the heart of London', suggests the internet. That's the ticket, so I buy a ticket.

'Right, how are we all doing?' says David, an ex-firefighter who will shortly be zooming a small group of us, currently standing on Blackfriars Pier in life jackets, up and down the river. The sunshine is scattering fairy lights over the gently rippling water, the murky old oxtail soup of a river today resembling a sea of chilled Evian.

'Do you live nearby?' David's daughter Ruth asks.

'Yes, I live just up the road in Finsbury Park,' I lie, in a mockney accent. I wish I didn't keep doing this, it's a bad habit. I do it because I think 'I live in Godmanchester' will lead to more conversation, but then I could just say Cambridgeshire. It's a rude habit, and I dislike myself for it.

These are the only details of the boat trip I can really remember. I have selfies of me on the boat, grinning and giving the thumbs up, so I know I had a nice time, but my memory hasn't retained any of it. Blank. It's so hot. I took a taxi to Notting Hill to see the carnival, not realising it starts on the Sunday. I have pictures of me walking around the streets, but it looks like I'm not really there, like I'm standing in front of a green screen. My navy Hawaiian shirt adds to the surrealness; I look like some kind of poolside magician.

The next three days are spent in my bedroom at Tina's. I don't remember getting back here, and now I am here I can't seem to leave. I spend twenty-four hours without water before I complete the Mission Impossible to fill an old bottle in the bathroom. My mind is holding me hostage. I have some bread and jam in my bag, but I can't pluck up the normality of asking Tina for a plate, so I make a sandwich on the drawers next to the bed, using a loyalty card as a spreader and a T-shirt as a chopping board and place mat. There's no place weirder than the inside of a head. I spend far too much time in mine, because the exit door keeps disappearing when I need it most.

I start to lose the plot. I can't handle being here. I should have made a plan rather than attempt to freewheel. Get a grip. Lying on the bed, brain flickering like a bad bulb while the sun ups and downs, the sound of children screaming and clattering as they play outside, I'm convinced it's a hallucination it must be it must be just screaming and squealing but I can't look and my whole body oozes treacle-thick sweat that smells of old coins. I'm not sure how it's possible to perspire this much for this long. It all goes a bit Ralph Steadman. I am trapped in this room and my mind appears to be disintegrating and I will never leave this room I will always be in this room.

And then ... *click*.

I'm in an empty Indian restaurant with a saucy chicken meal in front of me. I'm not hungry at all. How did I get here? I fake a call from 'my wife' who 'needs me home' and ask for my meal to be packaged up, which I end up leaving next to someone sleeping on Tollington Park Road. I'm relieved to be outside. I think it's Sunday. A cool silk scarf of evening air wraps softly around my neck, mollifying me, as the wavering tone of a tuning fork hums inside my head. My eyes vibrate. Everywhere smells of barbecue and beer bottle tops. I feel like I've been on back-to-back long-haul flights, my brain stunned numb, zapped-out and empty. Absolutely zonked, I am. And as I watch myself walk down the street, I'm almost certain it's time to get myself home.

I feel like I'm back at square one, without even knowing what square one is, or what sort of square I'm looking for. Tina later sends a message asking if everything was all right with my stay, seeing as I was in the room so much. I tell her I suffer from anxiety and that it was particularly bad the past few days, not helped by the freakishly hot weather. She's understanding and we write each other nice reviews.

I decide to have a little break after my Finsbury Park experience. I need to get my head back together; I've not been feeling too stable. Mum, Dad, me and all the family sail from Godmanchester to Brampton Mill on the Great Ouse Ferry. It's a rather grand name for a modest and ramshackle but lovely boat skippered by Captain Tim, a good old chap, relaxed and crumpled, and friendly, but with a cantankerous sense of mischief and a seemingly optional deafness, who picks passengers up by the Chinese Bridge and sails them back and forth to the Brampton Mill pub restaurant in the waters beside Portholme Meadow (the universe's largest water meadow). It comfortably holds around ten to twelve, if my counting serves me right, and is a most charming way to travel to lunch. It really suits Mum, too, as she's been unable to be a passenger in a car since a bad crash when she was eighteen, the seat-belt-less car flipping three times and landing upside down.

That reminds me, I nearly killed Dad in the car the other day. The driveway exits on to a blind corner. You have to edge out very slowly. It's treacherous, really. I inched forward a bit in Bakewell to get a good view and saw a car whizzing round the bend. In a panicked attempt to reverse my bonnet back, I managed the opposite and lurched further into the road. Somehow the oncoming driver swerved in time to avoid ploughing into us at 40 mph. 'Like I said the other day,' Dad states calmly, 'you ought to get a will done.'

It's a very pleasant way to travel, on Tim's slow, meandering boat. Much more my speed compared to the boat on the

Thames. And my family is much more my crowd than a load of tourists. My nephew Finlay tells me about what he'd been up to while Lisa, Pete and Freya were on holiday in France. 'I had my narcoleptic friend Louis over for a sleepover,' he said, casually. 'It got to about 4 a.m., Louis was asleep, obviously, but I couldn't sleep, so I went downstairs, lit some candles and ate a whole cheesecake. I just thought, "When am I going to get the chance again, you know?" so I did it.' He pauses in contemplation with a faraway stare. 'I don't regret it.'

I think about this the next day as I'm standing in front of the fancy boxed desserts fridge in Tesco at lunchtime, staring at a trifle so large it seems to be expanding with the universe. I'm remembering when Juliet saw a drunk businessman at Liverpool Street station devouring a whole one with his bare hands, when what appears to be another businessman stands a bit too close beside me. Maybe it's the same one. Maybe I've conjured him. Have I accidentally said 'trifle' five times in the mirrors of the chiller cabinet? This tall yet spherical gentleman with bloodhound eyes and a rumpled suit fitted like a tarp over a mound of sand picks up a family-size sponge cake and a pot of custard, looks towards me and in a deep bassoon voice says, 'Hehe, why not, eh?' Then just like that he's off round the corner and out of my life. I see him again at the self-service checkouts, fighting his cake and a Ribena Light into what seems to be a troublesome carrier bag. I like to reset my mind, after I've nearly lost it, in a supermarket. I find it comforting.

I need some handwash – one of the flavours is gin; who wants to make their hands smell of gin? – and out of habit more than hunger I put a sandwich in my basket. I buy some more cans of Diet Coke for my parents, who like to keep a large stock of them, and also Sprite Zero, in the shed. Oh, and I need to pick up another sack of kindling for the fire. A lady spills a load of cherry tomatoes on the floor. 'Oops, careful!' a man says, even though it's already happened, and I help to pick them up, while some shoppers are happy not only to just sidestep the situation but to actively walk over and ON the tomatoes. Psychopaths. No doubt the same sort of monsters who get on beds with shoes on, or tell off other people's pets. My sandwich, eaten in the car in the car park, is nearly ruined after a lady catches my eye just as I'm at the apex of a massive, messy bite. Mayonnaise and shame run through me.

'Hello,' I say, bustling shopping through the kitchen door.

'More Coke?' says Dad. 'We've got so much Coke, Robert.'

'You always ask me to pick some up when I'm out.'

'I didn't know you were going shopping.'

'I'm sure I told you I was, we had a whole conversation about it. You said to pick up kindling.'

'Anyway, it doesn't matter, I can put it in the shed.'

Mum comes in and expresses delight at a bag of chocolate-covered raisins.

The rest of the week is relatively uneventful. Mum and Dad are putting the house on the market, so an estate agent, a Porsche Cayenne of a man, comes round to talk real estate. Someone's coming to fix the downstairs loo in a bit. The flush button has stopped working. Quite an integral part of a successful lavatorial experience, the flush. I prefer a handle, myself. Or even a chain! But you only seem to see those in either really bad or really posh rural pubs. It's all buttons now, or of course the unreliable sensors of airports and big pay-to-pee railway stations, where you have to wave to the wall for an hour before convincing it that flushing is a good thing.

Still, as long as it's a strong flush I don't really care. People with weak flushes, especially those who keep it quiet, can rot in Hell. 'I went on Amazon to research which type of button to get,' said Dad a few weeks ago. 'I nearly bought one that was a metre long! Massive great thing!' I can't get this out of my head, and I'm loath to research it in case it's not true and obviously just a misprint on Amazon. I just love the idea of a gigantic toilet flush too much to have the idea ruined. Imagine how hard it would be to press. You'd have to spin round and use both feet. Imagine the polishing it would take. There's nothing worse than a flush button with fingerprints on it. Last thing you want is two giant paw prints.

I arrive at the post office as it starts to spit, to deposit a couple of work contracts. Droplets stain the brown envelope as I pop it in the box and send Godmanchester's rain first class to London. It really starts to chuck it down by the time I'm passing the butcher's shop and rounding the left turn that takes you past Mark's house. Drivers turn their wipers to 'frantic'.

'It's miserable out there,' Dad says miserably as we stand guard against the weather at the living room window. Miserably, I agree that it is indeed miserable. We ponder in silence with miserable faces for a bit, reflecting on the misery of the miserable day. It's not even that miserable out there, but we're both happy to play our parts in the whole miserable production of forced British miserableness. He breaks the silence. 'I don't know, eh?' 'I know,' I reply. One day I shall miss these conversations. Everything is as it should be again.

29

Right. Here we go. Like a castaway having another go at getting his shoddy bamboo and plastic bottle raft, held together with frayed twine, through the breaking waves, I have yet another run at London. I thought about a month in Cambridge, but upon flipping a coin five times, London it was. This time, an entire month booked in a ground-floor flat in Kentish Town. I'd be fine if I was the sole occupant, yes, I'd be fine, wouldn't I? Healthy food, daytime spent walking for miles, evenings writing while perched on the little pink office chair in front of the desk in the living room. I have a magic lesson booked in Covent Garden, as well as a tea ceremony in Southwark. I'll get up to all sorts of Instagrammable scrapes. Yes!

No. Silly boy. Again I become trapped by myself and this time, completely unchaperoned, I can't resist the urge to drink. The trip starts off okay. I'm able to catch up with my friend Dan H, who's just moved to King's Cross. We did the psychology presentation I was telling you about together.

He was one of my ushers. You couldn't meet a nicer chap, and that's a fact, so there's no point even trying to prove me wrong. I was feeling optimistic, which should have been enough to tell me everything was about to go wrong. The tigers came clawing at my back, to quote Tony Hancock. I only have one drink, to begin with. It's funny how one quickly becomes two and two becomes twenty . . . it all expands more violently than the Big Bang.

Delirious dark days and days behind the curtains blend together. I only go vertical to collect my daily carrier bag from Camden Food & Wine, motorbiked to me by Deliveroo and slotted through the living room window, also through which a black and white cat occasionally comes to check on me. I'm far too scared to even contemplate using the front door, let alone going beyond it. It's dispiriting. A few times, on my way to another blackout – in an odd heap on the bed, unaware of which way is up – I find myself becoming not all that keen on the idea of waking up. It's unwise to fill your mind with poison: first drink goes down, and you can't believe how good you've got it; from the second one onwards, you can't remember a single decent thing in your life. I start to worry that this time, this too shall not pass. I know somewhere deep down, somewhere primal, that I have to get my raft back to the beach; I have to haul myself home to Godmanchester. If I stay here I'll end up in hospital, or worse: washed out to sea and drowned.

I work out later, through checking my train ticket receipts, that I lasted ten days in the flat. It felt like a day and it felt like a year. To cut this already too-long account short: reader, I got myself in a right pickle. I buried myself well and truly under the volcano. God knows how I made the journey home. No memory. The second half of September I spend at my parents, picking apples with hands that shake until October.

So, London was a mistake. I need to ditch this fantasy of taking myself away somewhere to romantically explore hidden gems on my own, before retiring to a room to read and write and think, like I'm Portillo presenting his show on trains. It never happens like that, and it never will until I sort out the issues in my head. You can't get away from yourself. I just end up in a mess, having a sad little nightmarish party for one. This time last year was spent in hospital, and I've very nearly performed an encore. A month in the bin. To paraphrase a great man called Douglas, I never could get the hang of Septembers. I'm still alive, though, which is fab.

'I need to slow things down a bit, I think.'

'I wish you'd stop going to London, it obviously isn't good for you,' says Mum.

'I know, I know.'

'You remember what the doctor said last year?'

'They all said a lot of things.'

'He said you won't win next time.'

All I can seem to manage at the moment, without having some annoying collapse, is picking Mum and Dad's apples and turning them into crumble. How to turn that into an adventure? Godmanchester Living Facebook page to the rescue.

Saturday, 12 October, 11 a.m.-3 p.m.
Huntingdonshire Community Plant & Tree Nursery
The annual Apple Day at the nursery in Godmanchester,
featuring lots of apples, and much more.

'Right, Mum, are you ready?'

'Do you think I need my wellies?'

'I don't know. Do you like wearing them?'

'Oh yes, they're comfy.'

'Might as well wear them then.'

'I'm just thinking, it's muddy down there.'

'Wear your wellies, then.'

'Good idea, I think I will.'

'Dad, we're off to the Apple Day, see you later!'

'What's he on about?'

It's really quite mild out, but we're well into autumn, so it's a legal requirement that we wear big coats. Despite the warmth, it's drizzly and dark, the sort of mauve day where all you want to do is curl up in a comfy chair and spill Custard Cream crumbs all down your cardigan. The sort of day when you just want to roast the hell out of a butternut squash.

We right-turn at the White Hart, heading down East Chadley Lane, past the postbox Dad used to use 'before they stopped the evening collection, now I have to go all the way to the One Stop shop!' Soon we're plodding by Godmanchester Baptist Church and the house where the two brown dogs – a Lab and a boxer – sit by the large metal entrance gates all day.

'Robert, do you have to walk so fast? I'm old!'

'Sorry. Does anyone go to the Baptist church, do you know?'

'It's packed on a Sunday, apparently.'

'Hmm … what do you think they mean by "apples and much more"? I wonder what the much more is.'

'Perhaps they have pears, too,' suggests Mum, as we stroll past the graveyard, which contains the stone: 'To the memory of Mary Ann Weems who was Murdered in the 21st year of her Age', and continue past the cherry trees and the cricket pitch towards the Godmanchester Community Academy, the little school that sounds like a police force. Apple Day is only a few steps further on. Someone jogs by on the grass. Oh yeah! I was going to do Parkrun, wasn't I? Two a month. Maybe next year. And I was going to run 100 miles. Ha. Because the period of life when I was running long distances was when I was happiest. I imagine it's very tricky, running into the past, no matter how many miles you cover. They haven't developed a running shoe that advanced yet. I'll kill that idea for good. No more extremes.

The nursery, which relies on a team of volunteers to help, is on a four-and-a-half-acre site and contains an orchard, nuttery, potager, cut-flower garden and vegetable garden. We crunch our way over the gravel to the first greenhouse we come to.

'Oh, gosh, please don't say that's it,' I say to Mum.

'Where?'

'That table in there.'

'Oh my god . . . Surely not.'

We try to stifle our giggles (we're not taking the piss like a couple of uncouth kids; unfortunately it's just tickled us) as we look at a trestle table upon which are scattered what I'd describe as 'some apples'. Not a lot of apples, just a modest spread of 'some apples'. Don't get me wrong, there's certainly enough apples to give you a bellyache if you ate them all in a day, which would be possible, but perhaps not enough to warrant a festival of apples. We stay by the table awhile and stare at the apples as if looking at the *Mona Lisa*.

After I've said 'wow!' about an astonishingly large garlic, and we've bought a bag of psychedelic tomatoes for a pound, all green and red and yellow, all nobbly and perfumed, we leave the greenhouse and trek a little further into the lovely grounds, over the soggy grass – squelch squelch squelch like walking on porridge – and . . .

'A-ha! This must be the main event, Mum!'

'Hang on, I'm just sorting out my hood.'

There are three men pressing apples, a tent showcasing a range of apples, an apple condiment stand where I buy a jar of crab apple and chilli jam wearing a little gingham hat, which I'll crack open when the Christmas cheese is wheelbarrowed into the lounge after a heated game of Pictionary, a few stands selling cutesy little wooden bits and bobs – little signs for mums obsessed with (addicted to?) Prosecco, etc. – and a man with a clipboard from the Wildlife Trust. He's standing under a little green gazebo, showcasing a modest table of literature, and an upright map of the area which makes me think of a general plotting an attack.

'Hi guys, would you like to know about the work we do?' says Nathaniel.

'Yeah, sure, why not?'

Five minutes later, I'm buzzing about nature and have signed up to a monthly donation. I could listen to this chap all day, so enthusiastic.

'Thanks so much for agreeing to that, Robert. As I say, if at any time you want to stop donating that's completely up to you, you can do that at any time. Could I just ask your date of birth?'

'Seventeen . . . eleven . . . eighty-three,' I say, with my neck crooked round towards his iPad. I don't know why but you always have to monitor the process when someone is inputting your DOB on a form.

'All the best people are born in November, Robert. You've got a year and a week on me.'

'Scorpio?' I say, despite the fact that I now know from Nathaniel's last comment that he must be a Scorpio, and also despite the fact that I don't much care for astrology.

'Yep, indeed!'

'Wahey, nice one!'

Nice one? Where did that come from? Mum's staying quiet under her brolly.

'That's great. As I say, we'll send all your confirmation through by post and email. You've got your welcome pack. So yes, hope you continue to enjoy the nature reserves. There's so much stress and pressure in the world, it's so nice to just get away from it all.'

'Definitely, it's a great thing.'

'I've had a bit of a tough time lately – a week ago I lost a friend, so I've been a bit down, obviously not as much as he was, but even just a short time out and about in nature just makes you feel ...' Nathaniel pauses, a flicker of sadness crosses his face, and then he lets out a big exhale.

Back at the ranch, I peel apples and Mum cuts them into a big silver pan. 'I'll go to the Co-op in a bit, Mum, and see if they've got crumble mix.'

I take four bags of crumble mix and dump them in front of the lady at the checkout.

'Hello. Just these, please.'

'Is that everything?'

'Yep.'

'Making a crumble?'

'Yeah, thinking I might do,' I say, opening my wallet, in which one of my gout tablets has dissolved, so what looks like cocaine snows all over my shoes. Great, can't come here again.

I much enjoyed Apple Day. I think I'll try to stick with

milder adventures from here on in. Especially considering the results of the London adventures. I need to do things that are less likely to result in near death. Clearly I'm not suited to solo exploring, not at the moment, so I'll stop my attempts at that. My favourite escapades so far this year haven't been about locations, they've been about people. I suspected this would be the case (d'uh!); even the most basic motivational poster or Disney film tells us this all the time. I keep trying to run away from anxiety but it follows me everywhere I go. Almost like it's in my brain. Strange places on my own suffocate me; familiar people make it easier to breathe.

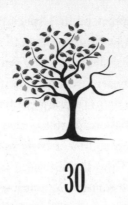

30

Hunter S. Thompson went to Las Vegas in search of the American Dream. B and I are in search of the British one, so we've come to Cobham Services on the M25, named by the *Daily Mail* as 'The Ritz of motorway service stations'. It's the busiest service station in the UK (I can hear your sharp intake of breath from here).

Interesting fact: tell people you're driving a couple of hours to visit a service station and that it's the sole purpose of your journey, and they will simply refuse to believe you. You'd have an easier time convincing someone you're off into space to eat the moon.

I love service stations. Not because they have all sorts of people there ('from pauper to prince, the humble motorway service station is the great social leveller, a mini cosmos of ...') but because they have loads of different types of burgers, and also coffee and seats and toilets and shops and sweets and stuff! The Cobham one even has a launderette – good for travelling hitmen. Granted they're not much to look at ... kind of a giant toilet, a huge baby changing area, a big off-white hollow blob, a vast vending machine ... but still good. You can't help but feel a bit of a kid in a service station, especially if you're already a man-child like me. And they make you feel like you're on your way to somewhere, because usually, if you're normal, you're in a service station because you're literally on your way to somewhere. Which is exciting enough, but throw a KFC into the mix ... holy moly. And you've gotta go there to come back, and when you do come back, hanging out of your arse on New Year's Day, the service station is there to wrap you in a warm greasy hug and fill you with nuggets and full-fat Coke.

'Oi oi!'

I'm sitting in my car, between Junctions 9 and 10 on the M25, in one of Cobham Services' 4,620 parking spaces, and B has serendipitously picked a spot mere metres away. He's walking by right now! He's an hour later than me because of an accident on the M25 – who would have expected that to happen? – which I just managed to miss, despite being slightly delayed myself due to having to fuel up at Toddington Services. It's the first time I've ever had to stop at a petrol station on my way to a petrol station.

'Oh, 'ello, sorry I'm late, you been here long?'

'Nah, just got here myself.'

B's come from his house in Leytonstone, but most of his journey time has been spent on the last mile of motorway.

'T?' (That's me.)

'Yeah?'

'What the hell are we doing?'

B is the man to call if you've got a madcap caper on the cards and you need a co-pilot. Modest, unassuming, calm and creative, he's the definition of having a good head on one's shoulders. A head with a shock of red hair, so red it caused someone in New York to actually shout, 'Hey, Red!' at him while he walked down the street. Like nearly everyone I know, he works 'in Content' and is the only person I know married to Vicky. Couple of legends. I was best man at their wedding. Yep. Did a speech and everything. B is the angel on my shoulder who I picture whispering, 'Just don't be a dickhead and it should be fine,' when I'm in a pickle and wondering whether being a dickhead will help. He likes chicken on pizzas, but nobody's perfect.

Cobham Services has a Pizza Express. And a Nando's. I've never been more excited to see either of them (especially with the recent rumour that Pizza Express is 'in trouble' – a rumour that's troubling us both beneath our stoic facades. Fingers crossed it's just some kind of sick joke, else I won't have anywhere to eat) as we strut into rest stop paradise. Note: if you've met up with a friend and you're all giddy and on the verge of hijinks and you're in a place that immediately requires walking off somewhere, like, say, a car park, then only the strut style of walking will do.

'Wow! Well, here we are, B! The Ritz!'

'Yeah! We're really . . . here!'

'It's a lot like the other service stations.'

'Sure is.'

'Shall we have lunch?'

'Yeah!'

'They don't have a Burger King, by the way.'

'I noticed on the sign. Ah, well.'

We narrow down the vast choice to a shortlist of two: McDonald's and KFC.

'Which is less busy?' asks B, as we scan between the two.

'Well, McDonald's has the order boards. Might be quicker.'

We're both huge fans of the order boards. Let's do this.

Waiting for our Big Mac meals, with arms folded and heels rocking, we chat about running. We used to do half-marathons together, really getting into the whole scene about five or so years back. We did the Royal Parks one twice and would train in Hyde Park after work. B tells me about someone he knows who smashed our half-marathon records without doing any training, an act that never fails to exasperate us.

'Christ, what is wrong with these people?!' I say, causing the customers waiting in front of us to turn around and glower at me. 'I mean . . . I can't believe how fast people manage to run without training! What is wrong with *those* people!' I continue, a bit louder, in an attempt to explain myself to the glowerers.

'Right, done that,' B says, as we sit at a counter with wireless phone chargers ('ooh!') sweeping shreds of Big Mac lettuce (did you know, the Big Mac was originally called the Aristocrat? Yeah, I know, pretty good fact) off our legs. 'What do you want to do now?'

Out the back there's a small lake with, as far as we can tell, one koi carp, some decking and a mini woodland trail. The building looks like a university library from this viewpoint. There's a sign by the lake stating 'No Fishing'. It's quiet back here. There's just one man giving his dog a stretch (walking it around, not stretching it like you'd stretch Stretch Armstrong). The car park and indoors are buzzing with Saturday travellers and coaches of Man City fans on their way to Crystal Palace, but it's a sanctuary out here.

'Does that sign mean someone actually tried to fish here?' I ask B.

'It's hardly a fair fight, is it?' he replies. 'A single fish in what's essentially a big pond.'

'Yeah! And look at that bin! Does it really need a McDonald's ad on it? Does everything need branding? Eh?' B laughs politely at this and changes the subject. When you're with a friend who you talk with almost exclusively in observational comedy quips, occasionally you'll bomb. We agree it's time to hit the casino.

I've always wanted to beat the house. In Vegas on a work trip back when I used to do exciting stuff, I put $60 on black. I lost. In a casino in Thanet on B's stag do he put a similar amount on black and cleaned up. He's my lucky charm today. We stay for one game of digital roulette and leave 80p richer ('Daddy needs a new pack of polos!'), thrilled to be rolling multiple adventures into one. This service station truly is where dreams are made. We retire to the massage chairs directly outside Quicksilver (in 2012 they became the arcade supplier at all Extra service stations, replacing Namco). Only my big black dusty pleather chair is working, so I spend a minute grimacing as my spine gets pummelled by this angry furniture. I'm almost certain the chair is trying to get information out of me. 'WHO SOLD YOU THE GOLD?!' 'PLEASE, CHAIR, I DON'T KNOW NOTHING ABOUT NO GOLD! ARGH!'

We regally cross the forecourt, taking in this den of debauchery, sauntering through this spaceship of sensuality, which is remarkable for me as I no longer have feeling in my legs, towards Starbucks. We're not so much here for the coffee, but for the layout.

'Shall we get some of that sweet mezzanine action?'

'B, you read my mind.'

We queue for coffee and play with the mugs for sale, banter

just streaming out of us ('Look at these mugs! Ha! Bunch of mugs').

'Did I tell you I used to work in a service station?' B asks. 'Back in Newport Pagnell when I was sixteen.' Our arms are folded again. 'I asked my supervisor for help with something, he came over and helped me then went back to scratching "fuck off" into the coffee machine. Then I burned my hand on one of those panini grills trying to push it down and had to go home. Made me realise I wasn't as clever as I thought I was. Quite a first day.'

'That's mad.'

'Then I was in charge of doing the cooked breakfasts, which was just loads of truckers having a go at me for not being able to fry an egg properly.'

'Nice.'

Sitting on the mezzanine, we survey the food court and feel like all that the light touches is ours. The Regus, the El Mexicana, the Tossed salad bar, the Harry Ramsden's . . . ours for the taking/using. Extraordinary. I show B a clip on my phone of a man dressed as broccoli getting arrested as part of the climate change protests. We spot a chap sitting with two whole roast chickens in the seats near McDonald's. We take some photos and then worry it looked like we were taking photos of a Chinese family at the next table while laughing. A restaurant meal, a casino, spa treatments, coffee . . . ooh-de-lally golly, what a day.

By the time we're in WHSmith's, and approaching expiry of the allotted three hours of free parking, even pointing at items and laughing is starting to wear thin. No words need to be said for us to realise this adventure is reaching its end. Our serotonin tanks are empty and we're running on fumes.

'Ha . . . look . . . a packet of wine gums.'

'Ha . . . yeah . . . Right, I'm gonna call it. What are you doing for the rest of the weekend, T?'

'Nothing. Just this.'

I've had more fun in three hours in a service station with B, and more fun on a bench with Chris in Godmanchester, than I had in four days in Barcelona on my own. You don't need a degree in larks to know that means: Mild + mate = yeah! Spicy + alone = meh! I get home to discover that we were unbeknowingly right next to an area of outstanding natural beauty in that service station. As beautiful as a Pizza Express? I doubt it.

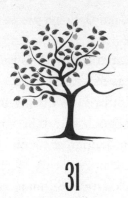

31

'ROB!' Juliet's voice flies determinedly over the Hammersmith Road to Suzu House. It's a mild midday Sunday in October and we're arriving here to make sushi. To attempt to make sushi, rather. Gorgeous platters of the stuff from the restaurants around Juliet's Soho offices are always popping up on her Insta feed, so this adventure is right up her street.

Juliet has steered me away from numerous unnecessary mini breakdowns – I take my toilet books very seriously, it's vital people laugh throughout their bathroom experiences, no matter what they're going through in there – and she works harder than anyone I know.

It takes a while for her to get the all-clear to cross the road towards me, so it's tricky trying to work out the optimum moment to say the secondary, closer hello before the final hug hello.

'Hey, how was the book fair?'

'Really good, thanks. Busy. I felt very responsible, being in bed early. So many people stay out all night in the bar. I just wouldn't want to do that, the days are so full on – meeting after meeting.'

'I saw you say you had a bad cold, as well?'

'I did, it usually happens after the fair. I've still got it now, but I'm fine. How are you? How's the writing going?'

'Yeah! Yeah, yeah, not bad, well, it's ... it's going, I suppose, is the main thing, so yeah, all good.' That'll convince her.

Juliet only got back from Germany yesterday and has schlepped here from Peckham this morning. She looks fresh as a daisy, ever stylish in a vintage coat and Halloween jumper. I, on the other hand, have had a week that only involved going to a service station and, standing here dressed in my navy outfit, look shagged. It's strange to be back in London after what happened. I felt a bit nervous coming here. Like returning to the scene of a crime. I've had no thoughts of extending this adventure into a full-on trip, though, it's: in, sushi, out again. Not every little thing has to involve a sleepover. Back home in time for the football. The one slight problem, however, is I'm a bit full.

Arriving on the Piccadilly Line ridiculously early, I've already had a main course breakfast at McDonald's, where hordes of delivery men waited in helmets to collect hash browns for Hammersmith hangovers, and where the faulty lights strobed and had me worrying I'd fit and die into my barbecue sauce; followed by my dessert breakfast in Costa, as bright and cheery as a 1970s snooker club. Someone smiled at me while I was having a coffee, so I've spent the past hour wondering if there's something wrong with my face. All of this fun took place in the shopping centre attached to Hammersmith tube station, which has the feel-good factor of a gigantic MRI machine. Come to this mall on a Sunday morning for the unbridled joy of leaving it.

I'm anxious about the sushi-making. I'd like to know how many people will be there, how interactive will it be, will there be a competitive element, will there be any sort of performing involved, will we get attacked by polar bears, etc., but all that is outweighed by looking forward to catching up with my friend. Juliet found the class on Groupon. I like Groupon, it's so enthusiastic. It's always popping up on my phone and calling me a VIP. Not all the offers are as fantastic as today's, though. Groupon's basically the app version of Del Boy. 'All right, pal, *mais oui, mais oui!* You look like a VIP sort, tell you what I'll do, I'll give ya 10 per cent off a spa day, but you have to go on a Sunday by yourself, now I can't say fairer than that, these tickets are like gold dust, my son, you know it makes sense. Lovely doing business with you. Oh, by the way, it's in Grimsby. Why do you think it's twelve quid?'

'Do you think we should go in?' I ask Juliet.

'I don't know, shall we?'

'Hmm, I'm not sure.'

'Let's see.'

We edge towards the door as if it might explode. It doesn't. Inside: a beautiful restaurant, clean and refreshing, like the smell of ginger at the counter by the door; quite minimalist in parts, yet still warm and welcoming, with back walls covered in pictures and tables set with colourful bowls and mats and chopsticks and cucumber, and pairs of blue food preparation gloves, a recent requirement from the good folks at Hammersmith Council. We're greeted by our teacher, the owner of Suzu House, Makiko Sano, who later tells the class that she studied at the Tokyo Sushi Academy, and take our pick of the seats at the very end of a main long table. We're the kids at the back of the bus. We busy ourselves with catching up as the room fills.

'How are your parents?'

'Yeah, good thanks!' I reply.

'I feel like I know your mum, we're best mates on Instagram!'

'Oh, she loves your Instagram. She's obsessed with your cats.'

At this point I'm in a battle with my blue gloves. Makiko, who has the vibe of those teachers in school who you really got on well with when you listened and engaged and impressed, but who you fear would have you over the rugby posts if you acted up. Well ... she's sort of started the class now, and I'm still dicking about trying to rubber up my fat fingers. Imagine trying to put on a pair of trainers a size too small over a pair of slippers while a tiger approaches; that's the panic levels I'm at. Then ... snap. I've ripped a glove. BUGGER. It looks like a spent balloon lying across my hand. BUGGER BUGGER BUGGER. I've ruined everything now. As I'm about to go home, Makiko kindly hands me and a few others a larger, sturdier pair of white gloves.

'I must say, this is very therapeutic,' says Juliet, as she takes great care in spreading sticky rice in an even layer over a sheet of seaweed.

'Yes, it feels a bit like being in playschool, doesn't it?'

'It really does!'

There's something quite adorable about watching a room full of adults (there are actually a couple of kids here today, who are streets ahead in terms of skill, knowledge and patience when it comes to the task of making maki, so I'm ignoring them and their gall) looking like determined but content toddlers, all furrowed brows and tongues sticking out of the corners of mouths in concentration, as if drawing a nice crayon picture of a kitty-cat. For now, for just a few hours, the grown-up world and all its tangled considerations is outside Suzu House and paused.

'The knife we use for cutting is very sharp,' warns Makiko. 'This one is not quite so sharp as I use, but it's still very sharp. When you clean it, make sure the blade faces away from you. A lady I was teaching recently held the blade the wrong way and ...' The mime that accompanies this story has us all pretty sure of the end. I know I won't be silly enough to make that mistake, I think as I cry my way through a mouthful of wasabi that I'm trying to prove isn't as hot as we've been told, but we worry for the person sitting next to us, who has so far appeared to suggest to us that she doesn't like sushi, doesn't like cooking, and is here by mistake.

The cutting part takes place at the head of the class and is rather on show, with only three of us allowed up at one time to chop our long rolls into bite-size morsels, so we both whack through it. I think Juliet and I are similar in that we don't like to mess things up and we like to please and impress (to a 'Monica from *Friends*' level), particularly with combining speed and capability. But with that comes anxiousness which, in this case, leads to ... 'WELL! Our sushi looks SHIT!' Juliet's not wrong. It's meant to be uniform in size and shape, identical in neat little rows. Ours looks as neat as Shane MacGowan's old teeth. We've made shanty towns of rice. 'We could always make it our thing,' I suggest, while urgently trying to eat the evidence of what we've done. 'Start a place called Wonky Sushi?' Juliet looks at our creations again ... 'LOOK at it, Rob!'

The two hours go by in a flash. It's been a ball. Everyone should do this. I'm back into 'it's good to do stuff' mode again, which often happens when I do stuff, but not always. As Makiko says on her website, 'In such a busy world, I believe that it's important to find time to take part in a craft, and perhaps learn a new one'. I suppose the bit I'm missing in life, aside from the busy part, is the 'learn' part. Must try to learn rather than just have a quick go.

I think about this on the train home. On the tube, Juliet told me she was going to qualify as a personal trainer, just for the love of it. I found that astonishing. I really lack commitment. I want better skin, but I can't be bothered with a routine. I want to know how a car works, but can't be arsed to lift the bonnet. I want to speak Spanish, but not enough to learn it, even with an owl willing to teach me for free. But why? Part of me blames a sort of pathetic teenage nihilism (is there any other kind?): why make a bed when it'll just get messy again? Some say alcohol freezes you in time, mentally, from when you first started to abuse it, so you can end up a teenager until you stop. And thinking about it, at the start of my teens I spent my time lying on my parents' living room floor watching *The Simpsons*. Yeah ... still doing that.

But this is just more reverse engineering, like with the eating challenge. Layers of excuses, like the layers of chub I can't be bothered to remove to reveal the stomach muscles I've always fancied. What's under all the layers? What's at the centre of an onion? Isn't it just more onion? Peel away the 'I can't be bothered because it'll just go wrong anyway' layer, and underneath must only be laziness and anxiety. But which feeds the other? Or are they one snake dining on its own tail? A snake ... eating an onion? Should those imposters be

226

treated just the same, like Kipling's Triumph and Disaster? Although they're not imposters like Triumph and Disaster, they're real and honest; innate. Worry and laziness: If I could get rid of one, would the other survive? Can't work it out. Head hurts now. Best not to think about it. Sorry about all the onion stuff. Be here now. Be here now on this train, where I can't open my takeaway box of sushi because I'll make everything smell of salmon. Never mind. I need to decide on my next adventure . . . something big. Something impressive.

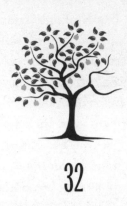

32

I've bought a yo-yo. It's red. I've also bought a yo-yo trick book, which is blue, with all the classic yo-yo showstoppers. 'Walking the Dog' – remember that one? Always wanted to have some kind of party trick. Shame I had to cancel the magic lesson; must rebook it. Yo-yoing is fun for about a minute. Not as fun as the fidget spinner I bought a few years ago. Raffy absolutely hated it though, so I stopped using it. I think I'll give this yo-yo to James as an extra Christmas present, it's wasted on me. Findings from finding myself impulse-buying a yo-yo: I really need to have sex again soon.

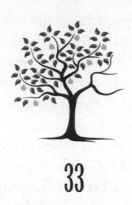

33

Right, it's time for a skincare routine. It's time for me to have
one. One that's routine. Good skin equals boosted confidence.
My face isn't too ruddy at the minute, so I'll concentrate on
body. My shoulders could do with a polish. How fine it would
be to have statement shoulders, waxed like a showroom car.
When I think of wellness, of purity and clear-headedness, of
sitting cross-legged in front of a big window wearing baggy
white linen and caressing a large rustic mug of something
hot, leafy and bitter, I think of Goop. It's synonymous with
the modern lifestyle rebranding of the word 'detox', which is
no longer just the job of the liver, kidneys and Librium, it's
also the job of body wash and, as we've seen, not looking at
phones. (Body wash and not using a phone are both suited
to showers. Maybe the shower is the best place to be? I'll live
in the shower.) 'Welcome to the world of wellness,' I say to
myself, as there's nobody else here.

I paid a friendly visit to the Goop website last week to
choose a few bits. The first product which caught my eye was

'"The Martini" Emotional Detox Bath Soak' (£30) which features Himalayan Pink Salt and Chia Seed Oil. 'There are three cups of bath soak in every bag – which means 3 [*sic: the Goop writers switch to a numerical three here*] amazing baths, all for you.' How kind of them not to insist on sending a Goop representative to join you in the tub. I decided against this one, although it sounds lovely – I imagine it would make one feel like being the star ingredient in a stew, or a big chunky olive in a cocktail – because as I've mentioned, I'm not a bath guy. Then there was the bamboo toilet roll at £33 for 24 rolls (don't let pandas near it, they'll gobble the lot: to them it's like a fat roll of delicious bacon). Not to bemoan expensive things, but just to deliver you a fair and balanced report: that's around £1.40 a roll. For the same price you could get about ninety Andrex. Or 300 rolls of the really cheap stuff that's like trying to mop up Nutella with tinfoil. Or you could just steal the industrial roll from work, or use sheets of newspaper – they're usually both of similar quality. If you're still reading, thank you. I'll repay you by moving swiftly on.

This luxe eco wipe is billed as 'clog-free' (personally I prefer the 'guaranteed clog' kind, but each to their own) and as 'toilet roll with a conscience'. Decent morals is the first thing I look for in a loo roll, to be honest, along with patience, wit, confidence and lashings of derring-do. Alas, I've just bought a load of Tesco's own, so there's no room in the cabinet for Goop roll (mmm, Goop roll ... sounds nice, doesn't it?). What else? 'The Sex Gel' (£20), a water-based lube that's 'cushiony'. Cushiony? I'm intrigued, but sadly I did a quick calculation based on recent coitus consumption (I can see the yo-yo looking at me) and concluded it'd likely sit in my bathroom cupboard longer than the weird tin of mussels has sat (patiently, I'll add) in the kitchen one (think it's been there since the signing of the Magna Carta).

I searched on. What was this thing? It looks like a razor. 'Gold Sculpting Bar by Jillian Dempsey' (£187). 'Made with 24-karat gold, it uses subtle vibrations to make the face appear more sculpted; it feels amazing, like a firm massage. Dempsey uses it to get her clients ready for the red carpet, but recommends using it daily for 10 to 15 minutes for optimum results'. Hmm, thanks to a pricey water leak at my house, I can't really stretch to £187 at the moment, so my face will have to remain unsculpted, staying in its usual blob shape. Plus I'm rarely on a red carpet, so it would be an extravagant purchase to say the least. Ah, AH! I thought, this looks more exciting, more adventurous. 'The G.Tox Daily Detox Duo' – two mentions of 'tox' in one title. This is the one for me. The two items included (£44 + £15 shipping) are:

1. G.Tox Ultimate Dry Brush: dry-brushing is an essential – and energising – skin-detox step. Made from pure, natural sisal, this brush exfoliates lightly and sweeps away dead skin cells to reveal glowing and smooth skin. Use it right before you turn on the water.

2. G.Tox Glacial Marine Clay Body Cleanser: this luxuriously creamy body wash is made with a hand-harvested glacial marine clay that's full of essential minerals. Together with nourishing organic safflower oil and cold-pressed moringa oil, it lathers into a rich foam to deeply cleanse while leaving skin feeling impossibly soft. A targeted, holistic blend of essential

oils – helichrysum, rosemary, grapefruit, and pepper-
mint – detoxifies and purifies.

Sounds dreamy. Sounds tasty. Sisal, I discovered via Wiki, is a sort of plant-based fibre. I feel like such a Luddite not already knowing that, as Goop seemed to expect of me. I've spent thirty-six years without doing any essential dry-brushing at all, and I have a coarse, acne-prone back to show for it. My usual shower routine involves taking a bar of Simple Soap (four bars for £1.25), thrashing it around me from head to toe, then spraying it off using warm/hot water. Although a delicate, honest, faithful and kind-spirited product, it can leave my skin feeling rather tight, like a guitar string tuned five octaves too high. Bending over to put my socks on makes me worry I'll snap and spring all around the bedroom.

To prepare for my new brushing routine, I read a Goop blog: 'How to dry-brush, and why it's so potent'. It begins, 'Stacked among the clear glass jars of homeopathic remedies, immune-supporting supplements, rose creams, and carrot cleansers on the sparkling shelves of the Organic Pharmacy on Bleecker Street in New York, you'll find a long wooden brush that looks straight out of an especially well-made Norwegian sauna.' Shall I check? How long would it take to get to Bleecker Street? I should probably just take their word for it. 'Especially well-made Norwegian sauna', I think, so not a bodge job Norwegian sauna made by cowboys you all too often see on *Rogue Traders*. 'Dry-brushing is one of those rare things that feels just as good when you do it yourself as when someone else does it to you'. After I've unraised my eyebrow, I find the info I'm looking for, a step-by-step guide on how to use the thing. To paraphrase:

- Start at the feet and brush up towards the heart
- Use small strokes or a circular motion
- Don't press too hard
- Three to five minutes of brushing, recommended in the morning

Add that five minutes of body-brushing to two minutes of teeth-brushing and ten seconds of hair-brushing and (hang on, iPhone calculator . . .) that's SEVEN MINUTES AND A BIT. Just of brushing! That's longer than it currently takes me to wake up, groom and eat breakfast. I can't wait to try dry-brushing when I'm a guest at someone's house. 'Hey, everything okay in there, Rob? It's just . . . you've been in the bathroom for a while,' they'll say, worried, quietly annoyed and bursting for a piss. 'Yeah, sorry, just got to finish brushing my thighs and I'll be right out.' I'm gonna need a bigger toilet bag. Maybe I could transport it in a violin case. I wonder what the etiquette is regarding public brushing. I've brushed my teeth in a service station before, but would I get in trouble for brushing my bum? I'll ask Debrett's. Come to think of it, *Very British Problems* Book One is consistently number one on Amazon in the 'etiquette reference' section, so if even I don't know the correct protocol, the regular common-or-garden dry-brushers of this green and pleasant land must be really scratching their heads (using a Goop head-scratcher?).

It's an extravagant spend, I know. But I'm living with my parents, I don't drink or smoke, my car's eighteen years old, I'm sprogless . . . Gotta have some treats, and interest in self-care is progress for me; I should encourage myself on this high-end grooming journey. Hang on, who am I justifying this to? Probably myself. Anyway, my first thoughts on my detox brush and fancy suds? They're brill. They came in smart navy boxes. At first I was a bit surprised at the stiffness of the brush: I was expecting something a bit more silky, but it feels more like a mini rake. A little painful, actually, though I have the feeling that proper deep-cleaning/grooming requires pain. Detox isn't pretty, after all. 'I suppose it's a bit like when they smack you about with leaves, isn't it?' Mum later suggests. After I brush my legs and lower back, I have a pleasant burning sensation, much like with Deep Heat, and feel a little spaced out, which I'm a fan of.

I've done my shoulders and am about to step into the shower (intrepid journalism, this). I had my doubts but oh, it feels so good. Almost masochistic. Flagellatastic. I reluctantly step out of the shower feeling clean, though a bit indecent, but in a smug way. My shoulders are shiny like a wet dolphin! It reminds me of the feeling I had when work sent me to have a wet shave (for an article, not just because they thought I could do with a tidy-up) at Geo. F. Trumper in Mayfair. James Bond's barber, you know? I walked out of that salon a king, face tingling with the double-cheeked slap of chilly air, and acted upon a sudden urge to buy some expensive leather gloves. The shave didn't work alone; it was the decadence and the pampering that shifted my thinking for a bit. The shave was without question the closest I've ever had, but being very hairless on my chin isn't something I'm particularly bothered about. It's the experience and theatre of it all which gave me a rush; the ritual, akin to when you go somewhere posh to eat and the waiter debones your fish – somehow it makes it taste better.

Although the shaving adventure didn't go completely without embarrassment, of course. I'd been having a problem with my skin at the time. Some sort of stress-induced eczema. The doctor had given me some steroid cream to use sparingly, so naturally I plastered it on, which resulted in my face turning bright red and, in places, greenish-yellow. I even got some days off sick because of it, 'my face is yellow' being added to the list of ridiculous excuses that included 'I've painted myself into my bedroom' (Nigel) and 'I'm locked in my garage' (Mike). I'd resorted to wearing a light foundation to even things out a bit. What I didn't realise was that the barber would be wrapping my chops in a freshly laundered hot white towel. When he unwrapped me, I knew the towel would have now turned terracotta. Being the consummate professional, his only reaction was to pause for a fraction of a second as he saw the staining on his flannel before discarding it, but it was enough of a hesitation for me to notice. Mortified, again.

I'll go back to Mint Source when the posh wash runs out, unless I start coining it with the *Very British Problems* merch sales, but I might ask for fancy soap for Christmas. Some people see expensive grooming products as snake oil,* but as the twentieth-century philosopher Sheryl Crow said, things that make you happy can't be all that bad, or something.

---

* Snake oil – that is, oil from the Chinese water snake – for all the bad press, is actually rich in Omega-3 acids which help reduce inflammation. And while we're on the subject, I'm pretty sure the snake in the Bible was just worried about Eve getting enough vitamin C. Give the snakes a break, people.

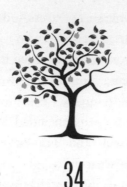

34

'Have you seen the fog, Robert?'

'Where?'

'Outside.'

'Oh. Yeah . . . well foggy.'

'Terrible. I wonder if everyone's got it.'

Mum and I are peeling apples and chatting about the fog while staring at it through various kitchen windows. Doesn't matter which angle you look at it from, there it is. It's so misty I expect a gorilla to dart across the lawn, not that we'd see it.

'We always get a day like this in October,' says Mum.

'Yeah, like the one that messed up my driving test! Then I couldn't take it again until Christmas, remember?'

If you live in the countryside you'll know that that's two whole months of possible McDonald's (bloody hell, my life really is sponsored by McDonald's . . . are you controlling me, McDonald's? Am I your Truman? Release me!) adventures ruined. My eventual tester, a man in black shades called Steve who dressed like an agent in *The Matrix*, directed us straight into a queue of festive shoppers trying to drive to Queensgate car park. 'Right, that's the end of the test,' he told me. 'You failed to indicate at any point, and that, technically, should mean you've failed, but I'm not going to fail you for not indicating.' What a dangerous but nice man. Luckily I have no driving planned today; today is all about walking. It's Halloween week, a holiday I've always either ignored or been afraid of, depending on where I was living and the likelihood of the door being knocked. Not this year: this year I'm going on a ghost walk.

'You waiting for the bus?'

'Yes, mate.'

'Should be along in a minute.'

It's a nightmare parking in Cambridge so I'm going on the X3. It's usually empty on the way in, and an empty bus is basically just your own big fat limo for a few quid. I'm at the bus stop on Tudor Road, having a one-way conversation with a chap who's gone a bit deaf. Well, I assume he's 'gone' a bit deaf because he's not a spring chicken, but he might have always been a bit deaf. Actually I'm just assuming he's deaf because he's ignoring everything I say back to him, but he might just find me really boring. Bus is taking a while.

'You go abroad and everyone talks to each other on buses, trains and whatnot, you know?'

'Whereabouts ... like, America, or ...?'

'Here we just sit in silence like dummies. We're the only country that does it.'

'Ha, yeah, it's very British, isn't it?' He has no idea how on-brand this conversation is for me.

'Trouble is, we think too bloody much.'

'Do you live in Cambridge, or ...?'

'Should be along in a minute.'

I'm not sure when to ding the bell. Outside the window is just a thick duvet of grey. At some point the sun sets, having never convincingly risen. The clocks went back yesterday, so Britain currently can't believe how dark it is. 'I'm sure it wasn't this dark last year,' Mum noted. Can't see a thing. Must be what it's like being in a submarine. In fact . . . yes, it reminds me of being up the Blackpool Tower. It's comfortable, here. Bumpy and warm. Eventually there's congestion and an increase in traffic lights. We must be more or less in the city now. I throw the dice and end up alighting outside The Punter on Pound Hill. From here, my new iPhone with its fancy ways tells me it's about a quarter of an hour's walk south-easterly to the Guildhall in the Market Square. It's here I'm to meet Tim, who runs Guide & Peek Cambridge, specialising in walking tours of the city. There's so much cleverness around, mostly dinging past on bicycles, that I'm positive just breathing in deeply buys me a handful more brain cells. Everywhere's so pretty. I'd love to live here. Pricey, mind! I wonder if I could wangle my way on to a course here. Something easy. Toilet Book Studies, perhaps.

Tim, who was once a student at Cambridge, emailed to say we'll be able to recognise him by his red hat. I wonder who else will be on this tour, which promises 'ghostly colleges, haunted bookshops, creepy alleyways, pubs with spirits and terrible puns'. If it's a big group, it doesn't matter, I don't have to talk to anyone; I could just pretend I don't speak English. Or I could just not speak to anyone, melt into the crowd, why would they care? I bet I'm the only one there solo. I nipped into a pub for a wee about ten seconds ago and now I need to go again. Perhaps I could just not turn up? No, that would be rude. If it gets a bit dicey it'll be easy to just peel away from the tour, claim in an email later that I lost the group while taking too long over a photograph. Yes, that's a good plan. I do a tour of the Market Square to scope out the joint. There it is ... the red hat. That must be Tim. He looks remarkably like Stephen, from the bee adventure. About ... four people around him. Right. One more loop and make my approach. Here I go. They've seen me, I'm now close enough that they know I'm one of the ghost walkers. Here we go ... committed now, for the next hour. I'm only a few steps away arrrrgggghhhhhhh ...

'Hello! Tim ... is it?'

'Yes ... hello! You must be ... Rob?'

'Yes! Hello, hello, hi, all right?' I say to the others, who are here from Connecticut with their daughter, who goes to the university.

'And you're from Godmanchester?'

'Yes, that's right.'

'Is there any special way to pronounce Godmanchester?'

'I'm not sure.'

'Because I saw something that said ...'

Just then we're joined by a couple, also visiting their daughter, from North Wales. 'Hello, hi, all right? Yeah.'

We wait a few minutes for the last few people, breath billowing into the fog and performing 'I'm cold' stationary hopping and hand-rubbing, and then we're off. I hang back, but from this point on, the pressure's off. I'm in 'being taught' mode again, my favourite. Gentle walking mixed with lovely warm historical facts and ghostly tales. This is easy. I think if I were a billionaire, I'd hire someone to just do a tour wherever I was going, even if just to the shops. A person to walk alongside me and describe the surroundings and their history. A human Wiki.

Have you ever noticed the lighting at night in central Cambridge? Walk along St John's or Trinity Street and look up and you'll see the Richardson Candles. Designed in the 1950s by architect Sir Albert Richardson, who hated modern street lighting, these elegant, wall-mounted tubes give off a haunting glow, similar to lamplight, which through the fog makes everything a sort of pleasantly punch-drunk sepia. In the gleam of the candles Tim stops us across the road from the terrifying crunch of the Corpus Clock, the Chapel of St John's College standing at our backs.

'Now, you see the creature on top of the clock?' asks Tim.

'Uh-huh,' some of us reply at various volumes.

'That's known as the time eater – he's actually eating up all the time we have. At the back of the clock, there's a small coffin with a clanking chain which tolls the hour. Now, the clock is only entirely accurate once every five minutes, to signify how sometimes time passes slowly, and sometimes it goes quickly. There's also an inscription, that translates as 'the world passeth away, and the lust thereof'. Now, us older folks, you know what that means. What do you reckon?'

Silence. Just before I'm about to say 'the older you get the less sex you want?' Tim says, 'The older you get, the less you care.' I'll be for ever grateful that the time eater didn't allow me a few more seconds to get my words out, else I'd be condemned to be mortified by this moment until all my seconds were up. I've never been more fascinated by a clock. Dad would love it.

My back keeps giving up on me as we walk, almost bringing me to my knees, so I make sure I'm out of sight behind the group to deal with myself quietly. Despite the fact that we're essentially just looking at streets and buildings, Tim spins a great yarn, and there are times I fully expect a ghoul to fly by or some demented figure to leap from the top of a church. The mist helps. Every alleyway would look perfectly in place in *The Exorcist*. It turns out Cambridge is bloody haunted. To put it in terms a lot less educated and erudite than Tim, bad stuff's gone down here over the years. At one point we're walking through a graveyard, I can't remember which college it's attached to, where Tim sneakily puts on the werewolf mask that's been sticking out of his pocket since the start of the walk. It's a charming addition to the fun. We walk by the Laboratory of Physical Chemistry – where inside there's probably a boffin in a white lab coat finely chopping up an atom, like garlic – bathed in spooky, pumpkin-orange light, and earlier we stood in a street that used to be an open sewer, where I was distracted by a young man in the flat above standing at the window smoking a remarkably large roll-up.

The last stop on the tour is The Eagle pub, where the graffiti of Second World War airmen is written on the roof and walls – 'Just think, for some men this would have been their last-ever drink,' Tim tells us – and where yer boy Crick announced that he and Watson had 'discovered the secret of life', which is not a bad day at the office at all. Imagine being mates with them.

'How are things?'

'Not bad. Uncovered the building blocks of human existence today. You?'

'I bought a slightly more expensive cheese than I'd normally buy, then I missed the bus.'

I say my thank yous and goodbyes and make my way back

towards the city's fringes. This has been a fine way to spend an evening. I'm buzzing again. Feel quite giddy, like when you leave the cinema at night after an exciting film and you think you're Batman in the car park. While I'm waiting for the bus home, outside The Castle Inn on Castle Street, a couple of chatting students stride by and one of them declares, 'I'm particularly interested in the military application of artificial intelligence.' There's the man who'll kill us all, I think. Bus'll be along any minute. Home for fish pie.

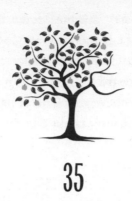

35

I'm in a Concorde. A stationary one, at the Imperial War Museum in Duxford with Mark and James. We've come to look at warplanes. Earlier this year it was the seventy-fifth anniversary of D-Day, and with Remembrance Day approaching and Godmanchester covered in poppies from roof to road, we thought it right to learn a bit of history.

My grandad Thomas fought in the Second World War. Mum's planning to take his medals to the service in town. He was sent a red dressing gown for his twenty-first birthday and wore it on parade, getting himself demoted for his trouble. He was a quiet, gentle man, who suffered from tinnitus and Ménière's Disease for the second half of his life. It's no surprise that we weren't allowed to talk to him about the war. It had broken a part of him. The mass graves at Belsen had done for his mind, and later on asbestos and Silk Cut did for his lungs, liver and stomach. He and my nan, Joan, who loved sherry and Wimbledon, lived next door to us when I was growing up.

Duxford is about forty minutes down the road, but I've never been. I went to the Imperial War Museum in Lambeth about a decade ago, to cover a Labrador called Sadie honoured with a bravery award for her work in Afghanistan. My memory wants me to believe that Cheryl Baker presented the medal, but it may be playing tricks on me.

'And?'

'James, stop saying that, please.'

'And?'

'Come on, eat your lunch.'

'And?'

'I wish you hadn't taught him that.'

We're on the M11 in Mark's VW Golf. The sun's extremely bright.

'Look, James, a cement mixer!' says Mark.

'Where?!'

'There. All the cement is being mixed inside that drum that's spinning round, you see?'

'Oh yeah!'

'I like things like that, that move and work while being transported. Like pigs being rotated on a spit in a truck.'

'Is that a thing?' I ask.

'Oh yeah, that's a thing. That's a thing, all right.'

'Like limousines with hot tubs on the back?'

'Yeah, like that. I like that.'

We park outside the museum and eat our petrol station meal deals (by the way, the Shell loyalty card is now an app. They scan your phone and you can pay for petrol on a credit basis. Thought you'd be interested) while James says 'And?' and we watch the planes manoeuvring on the airfield on the other side of the metal fence. A group of teenagers are outside the entrance dressed in army gear, part of their school's Combined Cadet Force (CCF). Mark and I had to do that at school, play army every Friday. We didn't have sex education, or anything at all relating to how to be a normal person, but at fifteen they taught us how to strip and clean a rifle. It hasn't once come in handy for either of us, as far as I know. My abiding memory of CCF was me, Jas and Nick getting sloshed on a bottle of Gordon's gin behind one of Stamford's many churches before marching practice. Jas and I got away with it, but Nick was swaying all over the place while attempting to stand to attention, and got suspended.

'Look, James! Bouncy balls!' We try one to check for proof of bounciness and it smashes all over the gift shop. We put it back and test out the pilot hats. After walking through a Concorde, gawping at guns, being spooked by dummies of soldiers – grotesque, slightly too large, somehow sweaty skin that looks like it has the texture of crème caramels – and caressing a fair few tanks in a hangar with that Jorvik Viking Centre kind of smell ('they're so solid!' we all agree), we have a break and a KitKat by a Spitfire. There's no food or drink allowed, but we decide these planes have probably seen worse. A father nearby is explaining to his young son that war 'isn't very nice at all'. I came here mainly for the adventure of trying the Battle of Britain flight simulator, but we're 20p short and they don't take cards, so we've no choice but to leave it. On the way home via McDonald's James is in full chatterbox mode, talking about his holidays in Southwold.

'Do you love it there?'

'Yes. The sand is just perfect! And when the sun warms the sea it's just so good.'

'Do they do nice food?'

'Yeah. The fish and chips I like especially. And they do Sprite and Fanta and Coke . . . all that good stuff.'

'Good stuff?'

'Yeah, you know . . . fizzy!'

'Fizzy's great, isn't it?'

'Yeah. And we play a game where the first person to spot the bridge on the way gets a lolly and I always win because I keep my eyes glued forward and everyone else is looking everywhere.'

Seventy-seven wooden soldiers were made to commemorate those from Godmanchester who died in the Great War. My mum has had one attached to the house, artfully framed, by her, with poppies made from the bottoms of large plastic pop bottles painted red and featuring black buttons in the middle, bought from a craft shop in Huntingdon. We ordered black pipe cleaners for the stems from Amazon. Not only has the wooden soldier representing Private Arnold Alfred, who lived on the street, been uploaded to the Goddy Remembers Twitter and Facebook pages, it's been placed on an interactive map featuring all the displays around town, from Crowhill to the top of Post Street, where the permanent stone memorial is. Mum, dressed in a beautiful black coat, carries the wooden soldier to the memorial for the service. She's been worrying about doing it right for weeks, losing sleep. 'Mum looks really lovely,' Dad says. 'I'm very proud of her.' Then morning halts, heads bow and everyone seems to run out of batteries as the town lets itself cry a bit. Sniffs, shuffles and coughs puncture the hush, the prematch throat-clearings like an orchestra's final rustlings before play. The A14 disrespectfully whooshes in the distance as Godmanchester concentrates on remembering. Birds keep chirping. We get home to find the soup maker has cooked us a nice vat of broccoli and Stilton.

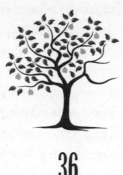

36

For my next trick, I'm going out for a sandwich. Christ, I love sandwiches. My death row last meal would probably be a Meal Deal. I've been sitting down, having a good think about what I'd really like to do today . . . about what would make me the most content, and a nicely made sandwich is the runaway winner. BL (Before London) I would not have considered this a plan in any way, but PL (Post-London) it seems to be on about the right sort of level for the good of my health. Aside from all the mayonnaise I intend to include.

It's garden waste collection today, and all the green bins are out, dotting the town like Monopoly board houses, but the hum of lawnmowering hasn't serenaded Godmanchester for a month or two now. It's past chilly, past brisk, verging on bitter. It's so cold you could store an egg on the pavement. I'm wrapped up, but it's so cool it's like my clothes are lined with cucumber. Dad's had to cover the bonsai trees. The waste lorry, wheezing like a smoker struggling to inhale every time it lifts a bin mouthwards, follows me slouching towards

Bellmans to be fed. In under ten minutes I arrive at the metal dreadlocks hanging in Bellmans door frame which, on this occasion, I jangle through with minimal embarrassment. It's a tiny place, hot and smoky from the bacon and eggs ever-present on the grills behind the high counter. There's a chalkboard of fillings and a baffling array of deal combinations and a tall glass-fronted fridge decked with cans of soft drink. As far as sandwich shops go, this one ticks all the boxes. I like it a lot. A couple of men in shirts and ties stand waiting for their orders. It's so poky you can't really get out of the way once you've ordered, so you symbolise you've been served by facing slightly away from the counter and looking at your phone. Get here really early, and there's usually a few uniformed policemen or paramedics, and blokes in high-vis, meaning that I'll order as if I'm in *EastEnders*. 'Awright, pal, bacon roll, ta ... eh? Oh, red sauce please, pal, nice one, diamond' (kill me).

'Yes, mate?' Two young women in the background, in white hats and aprons, prepare orders, scraping butter from industrial white tubs with big silver knives to apply to baguettes with one deft stroke, like plasterers.

'Awright, mate, erm ... I'll have ... sorry, are you being served?' You tit, I think to myself, you know the geezer in the tie's already been served, you recently saw it happen, and he's looking at his dog and bone! 'Okay, cool, erm ... can I have a chicken tikka baguette with coleslaw, ta. Oh, and a bit of salad, if that's cool.' If that's 'cool'? I knew I wanted salad from the outset, but I've tagged it on as a casual afterthought. And it's on the menu, of course it's 'cool', dude. Must stop saying cool, cannot pass for fifteen any more. Turns out it's not cool. As everything that's served here is always nice and fresh, ingredients are limited. 'Sorry, we're waiting for a delivery, no chicken tikka, no coleslaw, no baguettes.' Oh right, I see, I say, suddenly sounding much more posh, as if my brain is automatically gearing itself up to say, 'Now look here!'

'I can do you salad on a couple of rolls?' I must admit, while I appreciate the freshness of the food here, and am grateful for a proposed solution, it still rather knocks me for six. While I try to get my head around quite how two salad rolls constitute any type of rational substitution for what I ordered, days seem to pass. I can't just walk out. How has it come to this? Finally I utter: 'Yeah, cool. Can you do me a bit of mayo on those, too, please? Ta.' Can you do me? They can, and do. I walk out, with my two bread rolls filled with lettuce and tomato and a bit of mayo, the white paper bags quickly turning translucent with oil, feeling somewhat disappointed. There was plenty of other lovely stuff to choose from (they had non-tikka'ed chicken!), but I panicked. Arriving home, I find some chicken and coleslaw to add to my strange sandwiches. Maybe tomorrow I can go out to the cycle shop, buy some pedals, then rush home to build myself a bike around them.

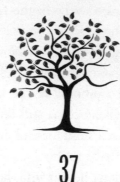

37

After half a year of mulling it over, I've decided that yeah, I'm gonna try boxing. I'm rising up, back on the streets, and my eye is now that of the tiger. Everybody seems to be boxing now. I wonder what they're preparing for – what haven't I been told? Lauren's said she'll show me the ropes. Although she refers to it as 'pad work', no matter how many times I say 'boxing'.

Lauren's temporarily moved from Bills Gym to a place called the Fitness Forge, around the corner. I make my mind up to try boxing and we've gone somewhere without a ring! Typical. The Fitness Forge is a big warehouse kind of place, with a large room upstairs – reminding me of the apartment Tom Hanks buys in *Big* when he gets big – mostly orange, with all the usual machines, and dance music so fast and loud that even the most hardcore UK raver would probably find it a bit much. Lauren puts on pads, I put on gloves, and immediately I feel quite embarrassed. Me, a shy, tubby writer, in boxing gloves, what an imposter! I'm also terrified of accidentally punching Lauren in the face, what with her head being right in between the pads and me having the coordination of a toddler. She doesn't seem too fussed about that happening, though, which says a lot for the weakness of my jab. She shouts out combinations, which my brain insists on thinking of as complex equations, causing me to repeatedly pause and apologise (something you don't see in a lot of boxing matches).

'Feet apart, steady, don't be too wild, keep it tight, snap it back in, remember to rotate that hand, your left's a bit naff but you're strong on the right ... good ... and again ... uppercut ... wrong hand ... you're doing well ... feet ... that's it ... rotate the hand ... okay, and ... rest.'

'Thank god for that ... Christ ... my wrists hurt. I'm absolutely shagged ... Christ ... let me just breathe for a bit ... dear me ... I'm dying ... how long was that?'

'That was twenty seconds.'

'Right. You can see why boxers have to be fit!'

'Yep.'

When I connect with the pad properly and it makes a loud smacking sound, like bubblegum popping, or a really well-executed high five, I get the same sort of buzz as when a tweet 'bangs' and gets a solid retweet from a high-number account, which is kind of sad, I know, but yeah, that's certainly the closest thing I can think of. Must be great to properly connect with an actual head, especially one that's been bad-mouthing you at the weigh-ins. Lauren runs off to see if she can get the music changed, while I go to scratch my forehead, still in gloves, punching myself in the eye. I can't get the lid off my water bottle. Quite thirsty. Hope Lauren comes back.

I arrive home to find Dad ripping cardboard into

playing-card-sized pieces, so they fit neatly into the blue bin that'll soon be tipped out into a big messy pile in the back of the lorry.

'Dad, if I bought a punchbag, could we hang it in the shed?'

'Erm . . . no?'

'Okay. Do you want me to take that cardboard down to the bin? I've already got my trainers on.'

'No, I'll go, I have to check the post as well,' says Dad. The postbox is outside, like in American films, near the bins.

'Well, just give me the key and I can do that too, while I'm out there.'

'Oh . . . really? Okay then, thanks very much.'

I shortly return to the kitchen empty-handed.

'I had a look but there wasn't any post, Dad.'

'No, we don't get post on Tuesdays.'

I'd quite like to carry on boxing, though Lauren and I are quite drastically different heights, so aren't really suited to being sparring partners. This means I'll have to find, oh no, some new hands to weakly wallop. I'll have to have a think about that.

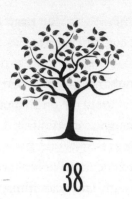

38

'Anyone in Cambridgeshire want to start a double tenpin bowling team with me? This isn't an impenetrable ironic joke.'

Send tweet. I've not sent a tweet like that before. Hope it doesn't look weird. Perhaps it does look a little bit weird. You have to say things aren't a joke on Twitter, because, if you happen not to have used it before, almost EVERYTHING on Twitter is a joke. Lots of stupid arguments as well. Arguments and jokes, often combined, are prevalent. Often you won't even know a tweet is a joke. But it is.

It worked! An artist called Chester, who also works a lot on social media, replied to me. Yes, he said, he would go bowling with me. I love bowling. When I lived in Stamford and worked on *Your Dog Magazine*, it was my only real hobby, aside from the pub. Nicky T, who worked in ad sales at the company, decided we should join a league. After work on Tuesdays, we'd get into our cars and race from Stamford to Peterborough to play in a doubles tournament. We both had monogrammed shirts – Bobby T and Nicky T – bought online for a tenner. Our team name was 'The Easy Ts'. Unfortunately, they entered it into the computer as The Fasy Ts, which doesn't mean anything, and made us feel quite ridiculous. We asked them to change it many times but they said it wasn't possible, making their computer surely the only computer in the world where you have just one go at everything.

Eighteen teams were in that league. Everyone else had multiple balls in huge bags. We didn't even have bags. Carrying our one bowling ball each in a sort of tea towel, we'd stroll into the arena and meet that week's opponents. I'd vigorously shine my ball, warm my hands on the little fan, then roll it straight into the gutter about twenty times. Then we'd leave. The manager even took pity on us and gave us a free lesson. 'I don't know what we're doing wrong,' Nick would often say, perplexed and dragging on a Marlboro Light. 'I think we're just bad at bowling, Nick.' It was the highlight of my week.

Bowling alleys seem to have gone multicoloured since then. After a stressful drive with lots of mini-roundabouts, I park on the ground floor of the Cambridge Leisure multistorey car park and walk past the IMAX, past Rocker's Steakhouse, which I've been in but can't remember why, and stroll into the does-says-tin-named Tenpin Bowling in Cambridge. Half an hour early, I perch on a seemingly abandoned bar stool among the arcade machines and busy myself signing up to the building's Wi-Fi. Then I just jump from Twitter to Instagram to Facebook and back again, not taking any of it in, concentrating purely on trying to look like a normal, relaxed human man. It's not a particularly relaxing atmosphere, though. I'm experiencing what it must be like to be trapped in a bag of Fruit Pastilles. The lights keep changing. Purple to pink to orange to purple to yellow to purple to green to purple. It's mostly purple, to be honest. Dark, as well. Like being in a whale's mouth. A couple of teenage girls play pool, but apart from that it's pretty much dead. This is my second attempt to get to this bowling alley to meet Chester, having aborted the first due to a bout of gastritis. He arrives, and we shake hands and begin pitching our personalities to each other. I'm not too bad with meeting just one other person; if he'd have brought a friend there'd be no talking from me, unfortunately. I'd retreat into my big warm shell. I can't believe I'm in the process of making a new friend.

'One Peroni and one Coke, please. Oh, and bowling, as well, if that's okay?' As the man behind the bar unscrews the cap of a half-full, two-litre bottle of Pepsi, pouring the warm, flat brown into a scratched-up branded glass, he replies, 'You can't actually pay for bowling here, you'll have to see my colleague over there.' He points to a till, at the same bar, less than a metre away from the till he uses to tot up the drinks bill. On my side of the bar, the two areas are separated by a single black rope the length of your average skateboard. It's easy, in the face of ridiculous rules, to be a bit openly snide about such silliness (oh the bureaucracy!), and though I like to think I've grown out of that sort of sniggering mockery, that I'm a nicer person (it's not this guy's fault, after all, he doesn't need some smart-arse comment, he's just a barman in a bowling alley), I think in reality I just can't be bothered with being snide any more. It's tiring. Hang on. Haven't actually said anything for some time. Must speak . . . NOW:

'Cool. Hey, Chester, thanks for coming, by the way, I didn't expect anyone to reply to that tweet.'

'Yeah, well, I didn't know if it was a joke or not, and if you just felt sorry for me.'

'No, no joke, although I thought it would be seen as a joke. That's why I said it wasn't a joke.'

'I thought that might have been part of the joke.'

'Yeah, I can totally see that. So much irony on Twitter!'

'My heating doesn't work at the minute, so it's nice to be somewhere warm.'

'I'm currently living with my parents for a bit – if anything, I've been too warm!' As I'm saying this, almost in tandem with the words coming from my mouth I think, 'Why would you tell a cold person that you're too warm? It's like telling a sad person that you're too happy. Stop. Don't overthink this, you wally.'

We round the rope in three steps and pay for two games of bowling. We're on lane five to start with, which breaks so we're moved to lane six. To the left of us, a family with lots of kids, to the right of us two teens, a boy and a girl, more interested in sucking each other's faces than getting strikes. Losers. Although, saying that, it's always uncomfortable, getting a strike; how the hell do you celebrate? Awkwardly walk back, smile bashfully and apologise? Or sink to your knees and punch the air? I'm the former. Turns out, with my form, I don't need to worry about this scenario too much. I've warned Chester I'm not very good at bowling and he's returned the warning. He wins both games. 'I'm so glad I didn't bring my ball,' I tell him. 'It's navy and has "Bobby T" engraved on it.' You try walking away from a lane carrying your own monogrammed ball when you've just bowled a sixty-eight; when on your first bowl of the night you fall over. I've almost always been embarrassed about owning my own gear. I think it stems from when I was at junior school and we were forced to play the recorder. Britain loves a recorder.

All my classmates bought the classic black plastic number in the corduroy bag, but Mum and Dad bought me a special recorder: wooden, in three pieces, in a red leather and velvet box. It came with a little pot of grease for slotting it together. A little pot of grease! Mortifying. 'Yeah, a ball is a big commitment,' Chester agrees. Look at me! Chilling out, bowling, shooting the breeze.

Maybe I'll become a bowling guy, maybe this was what I was meant to be. As a young man I wanted to be Bukowski, like all young men doing English Lit, somehow thinking that drunkenly living in a bedsit with stained underwear was glamorous, but I should've been striving to be Lebowski! I love dressing gowns, I love bowling, it fits. Granted, I'd prefer to do it in a more old-school bowling alley, rather than this Vegas Lite migraine palace, but I'll take what I can get. We play a couple of games of pool – 'You should've brought your own cue,' jokes Chester. Yes, I should have brought my cue, I think! – then, after winning a game each, or losing a game each, we say our goodbyes.

'So, do you fancy doing this again?' asks my new bowling buddy, as we shake hands outside. I get the feeling we're both not regular handshakers. We just sort of gently touch our palms together rather than shaking. 'Because I live nearby and I don't really . . . do a lot.'

'Yeah, that'd be great!' I blurt. 'I mean . . . same, really, I don't do much at all.'

'God . . . we really are internet men, aren't we?'

'Yeah. Yeah, we are.'

I get home to find Mum constructing a bowl of various sweets that's as pretty as a flower arrangement. I send Big Dan an early Christmas gift: a box of Ritter Sport Joghurt via Amazon. I find Dad in the living room watching a nature documentary.

'If we were more like ants there wouldn't be all these wars,' he says.

'How do you mean?' I ask.

'Ants look after each other,' he replies, sagely. 'They've done studies.'

A few weeks later I get in touch with Chester to ask if he'd like to go bowling again some time, to which he replies that he would, though we don't set a date for it.

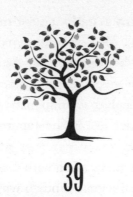

39

I've had a dream. Just woke up. If I may, I'll tell you all about it (fictional teenage lad Adrian Mole said the only thing more boring than listening to other people's dreams is listening to their problems, but if you've made it this far through the book then I'll assume you have a high tolerance for putting up with both). It was my usual A-level anxiety dream that I've told you about, but something extraordinary happened this time. I entered some warped version of my old school hall, and realised I was there not to take a test, but to receive my results. I was petrified, but not for long. Mrs Dobson, who'd taught me for one year when I was eight, opened her desk drawer, and in the manner of a GP said, 'I'm pleased to say it's good news,' and handed me a piece of paper. Three Bs. I hadn't revised for these exams at all; they weren't even in subjects I took at university. In fact, they were my worst subjects: maths, history and, in the dream, 'science'. Three Bs! Relief smacked me like the sweetest kiss. I actually woke up laughing! I've done it! Three Bs. I mean, that's a good result, isn't it? Funny how

I didn't give myself any As. Not that it matters. I'd expect at least one A, though. This is bloody typical of me: thanks, brain, you couldn't have given me three As, could you? Three Bs ... good, perfectly adequate, solid, unquestionably competent, more than enough to get into many a decent uni, who wouldn't be happy with three Bs without any revision at all? I mean, in the dream my answers are just gibberish, so what a turn-up! But even in a world of make-believe I still can't aim higher. 'You've done all right, old boy,' says my subconscious. 'But don't go overboard congratulating yourself, don't get too carried away, they're only Bs, it's not like you got As. Well done and all that, but steady on. Now, come on, I'll take you to Pizza Express for a congratulatory lunch, but no starters.' I should get out of bed, I've been thinking about this for half an hour now. My mind feels a little bit changed, fuzzy and damaged but not in an unpleasant way, like when you dream you're in love with a friend and wake up all confused, wondering if you should call them up and propose (reader, you should not).

I thought about trying rock-climbing today. Then I decided I wouldn't like it. After thirty-six years of life and a year of doing more stuff than I've done in half a decade, I'm starting to believe a 'don't knock it until you've tried it' mentality is, perhaps, sometimes a bust. I know I won't enjoy climbing rock walls. It's not for me. I knew I wouldn't like oysters. Wanted to like them, though. Tried them, willed myself to enjoy them, didn't enjoy them (I haven't a chance of beating Frank Skinner's description of eating them being like licking phlegm off a tortoise). And neither do you. You don't like wine or whisky, either, admit it (joking – don't write in). So going against every adventurer code there is, I simply won't try rock-climbing. Ha. The 'live each day as if it's your last, we'll all be dead soon!' eggers-on create a lot of pressure. That long film about the man in prison tells us to get busy livin' or get busy dyin', but what happened to get busy potterin' about? Some of my best days have been uneventful. Hey, maybe I'm learning to let go a bit. YOLO would be fine, if life didn't just keep on going; it's impossible to sustain; YOLOing makes me feel like I'm being left hanging on a high five for weeks on end.

Not everything has to be done against the clock. Take time off your mind. It's pointless to try to fight time; you can't win. And there's no use in trying to hide from it – it's a champion at seeking, it'll find you in seconds. So best to just let time get on with it, I think.

If today is proving tricky, it's probably not your last. Most of us have plenty of days. The idea that we (look at me, I'm on my soapbox now, I'm on a roll, I think I've had too much Haribo) have a deadline to 'get happy' seems counterproductive. Sack off today, see what tomorrow brings, and sack tomorrow off too, if you have to. Stay in your pyjamas. The only bad thing about wearing pyjamas all day is you can't look forward to putting them on. Like with drinking, though best not to do this for three days in a row. So, instead of being nervous on a fake cliff, Mum and I walk into town to look at Christmas wreaths in TK Maxx. We get a nice one from Thelma's Flowers in the end. I soon start to worry again that I'm not seizing the day. I blame motivational quotes for the rise of FOMO; they're not worth the cheap posters they're badly spelled on. Unless they do actually motivate you, of course, in which case: crack on.

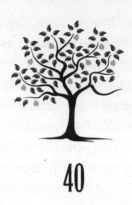

40

It's high time I joined the modern world. I need to stop settling for, and adapting to, the broken and update my life when the offer is there. I finally acquired a shiny new phone, placing my old phone, David, gently and respectfully in the wardrobe, and now I've only gone and bought a new iPad. Apple's new some-singing, some-dancing entry-level model, in my usual rousing colour choice of 'space grey'.

Once upon a time, back when tigers used to smoke, I was handed all my tech for free, what with working on a gadget magazine, but these days I have to smash open my piggy bank. The iPad I've been using for the past seven years would panic and freeze at the slightest request, would turn itself off whenever it felt like a rest and recently locked itself completely, so it was time to put it (Eleanor) out of its/her misery – wardrobe. All I use it for is reading and using social media in a slightly larger way, and now it can't even do those. It was also linked to my ex-wife's account, so I couldn't download or update anything, or link it to my phone in any way

(I'm sure all this information is fascinating you). And besides, nothing solves an existential crisis quite like shiny new stuff. As Hugh Laurie wrote in his novel, *The Gun Seller*, 'The only good thing I've ever noticed about money, the only positive aspect of an otherwise pretty vulgar commodity, is that you can use it to buy things'. I love Hugh Laurie.

I ordered it (still deciding on a name) online. The last bit of tech I bought in an actual shop was a big telly from John Lewis (or JL, as Chris G affectionately calls it). This involved standing in front of numerous screens in Queensgate, taking it in turns with the salesman, who for some reason was holding and occasionally swiping on a tablet, to say 'excellent' at really HD versions of *Finding Nemo*. Shaking hands on a TV that was twice the amount I'd budgeted for, I vowed never to shop for entertainment goods 'in the flesh' again.

Do you remember what setting up and syncing these things used to be like? Peeling off the protective layer of plastic (and keeping it in the box, for some reason); switching on your phone for the first time, being greeted by the screen – 'Hello!' – and then spending the next two days on the phone with customer support? 'I'm just going to have a chat with my colleague, Robert, is that okay?' 'Okay, Robert, I'm just going to put you on hold', 'Robert, bear with me, Robert', and then you're halfway through the *Back to the Future* trilogy before you hear from them again ... 'Okay, Robert, so I've had a word with my colleague and what I'm going to do is have him ring you back later if that's okay, is that okay for you, Robert? Okay, and do you have a number I can phone you on, there, Robert?' Not like that any more, is it? I've just turned on the iPad and it's done all the work itself. 'Ta-dah,' it seems to ding. This was almost too easy. Suspiciously easy. Unsettling.

Still, it's nice to know that everything on my devices is synced, my photos won't randomly delete themselves any more, that I'll have storage space for new things – I can stop reading the same four books over and over again! – and I won't need rubber bands to hold my phone (what is essentially my life) together. And it didn't take any time at all. I was worrying about upgrading for years, how much of a bother it would be, and it set itself up in minutes. All that worry for nothing. I also go to my laptop and clear off all the viruses and malware, download the latest OS, clear my desktop and buy a program which sweeps through my computer in seconds and frees up acres of space. I don't even know what it's deleted, but it deleted a lot! I've Marie Kondo'ed my gadgets. I should have done this years ago, dealt with all the crap rather than learning to live alongside it. I feel rather proud of myself. Achievement unlocked.

Something must be about to go wrong. It doesn't feel right at all. This isn't very me. Later that day I accidentally walk the new iPad into a door and break the power button. Aaah, that's better. Oh, and the exam dream's back, by the way. Hurrah.

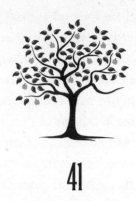

41

I'm walking down Cambridge Street in Godmanchester when I see a clinic I haven't noticed before, with a sign saying, among other things, 'Indian Head Massage'. Indian head massage. Hmm. Sounds nice. What is it good for? Let's ask old man Google. Indian head massage is said to encourage oxygen supply ('go on, oxygen, go on, you can do it, good lad') to the brain, reducing anxiety and helping you think clearly. Ideal. My neck's been stiff recently, too, especially when I wake up. You know you're getting old when oversleeping injures you. Conclusion: sold. Rather than just go in (what if they don't like the look of my head?), I go home and ring. 'Oh, I'm sorry, love,' the lady says, 'I'm afraid the person who used to do that doesn't do it here any more.' Wonder what happened. 'Okay, no worries, thank you anyway.' Hmm, someone must rub heads around here. Hello, Google, me again! Here we are, Adagio, on Huntingdon High Street, a stone's throw from the Cromwell Museum and Pizza Express, on the end of the road with all the estate agents. Appointment booked for 4 p.m.

This'll be a good chance to take a box of stuff from my house to Scope, it's in the same building as Adagio. Why's it called Adagio? Isn't that music? Google, what do you reckon? I don't think I go more than five seconds at a time without whipping my phone to my face. Ah, it's Italian for slowly, or 'at ease', very clever, like it. Mum's already packed up the box for me. She's spruced the house up; taken away some of my decorations and put up some pictures of parrots in the living room, which are 'all the rage'. The place looks great. Mum's a master of interiors and packing. When I move house, a typical box packed by me will contain a big pepper grinder, a nearly empty bottle of ketchup, five DVD cases with the discs missing and a saucepan lid. Mum could take a small box and fit the entire contents of Homebase into it.

Actually, I'll take the box tomorrow in the car, it's too heavy to walk with. I say bye to my parents, who are sitting in their places in the lounge in the dark, instructing each other to look at the rain, put on my big navy coat and venture bravely out for my heroic adventure of being stroked like a cat. It's stormy out, I feel like a sock in the washing machine. Pushing against the flow of schoolkids biking home through muddy puddles, the girls on the whole sensibly wrapped up in hooded coats, the boys occasionally flicking wet fringes out of their eyes but otherwise immune to the weather, I'm soon passing the apple festival venue (great times) and The Black Bull, speeding towards The Old Bridge Hotel on the edge of Huntingdon, the corpse of the old A14 hanging over the Ouse to my left. The footbridge tells cyclists to dismount, but they never do. The hood on my parka is nicely all-encompassing, like an old-school diver's helmet – I have to turn my whole body to check crossings as it refuses to face anywhere but forward. Huntingdon is damp and Christmassy, with trees netted up outside shops and lights holding hands from building to building.

Adagio is written on the door in a kind of calligraphic way, as if it's a brand of Authentic* Italiano Ice Cream. Climbing the steep, carpeted stairs, dripping as I go, takes me into a salon, ten minutes early. 'Hello, is it Rob? I'm actually ready for you now if you want to come straight through?' I don't get her name. It's Lauren, but I discover that via their website later. There's never a good time during the massage process to ask for a name. Left alone in the small, dim room to undress (or 'pop' my top off) and seat myself on an office chair with a towel wrapped around me at the chest (surely the most stressful part of a massage, apart from the actual massage: worrying if you're going to prepare correctly and not arrange yourself in some ludicrous way that they'll talk about at the office party), the masseuse re-enters and starts to knead me. I made sure to dry-brush my shoulders for the full five minutes before I came (I've been slacking at an average of two minutes recently), so they're extra-glossy. She asks me if I've any areas of discomfort. I don't tell her that my neck's been a bit painful since I sat in a massage chair during a day out at Cobham Services. A small stereo, like the one at yoga, plays chill-out songs, like the ones at yoga; those songs that take fifteen minutes to fade out and then leave too many seconds of silence before the next identical song takes fifteen minutes to fade in, so you have a brief period of hearing oils squelching and deafening nose-breathing.

I wonder what to have for dinner tonight. Oh yeah, we're

---

* Made in Milton Keynes

having penne. I should buy some toffees for Dad. We've got plenty of sweets, but he doesn't like 'those gummy things'. I wonder how Tori's getting on. I should check in on her. Remember that time you wrote an email taking the piss out of your boss and sent it to him? Of course you do. You'll never forget that. I should eat more fish. I wonder if I should do something this weekend. Might end up drinking. We'll see. I haven't had a burrito for ages. How long would it take me to sail to Iceland? I can hear someone talking next door. Walls are thin in these places. Not as bad as that massage place in Balham ... with the washing machine. There's a loud woman at the reception. 'It's for a gift, you see, he wants a massage. What's this one?' 'That's head, neck and shoulders.' Hey, that's what I'm having! Ha! 'Hmm ... can I add legs on to that?' Incredible. She thinks she's building a burger meal. 'Well, with legs as well, that'd be your full body massage.' I want her to ask how much it'd be for only one leg. Thinking about it, I wonder ... do you have to pay full price if you're missing a limb? 'Okay, I'll get him that one then. He just doesn't want his face done, you see.' I have to stifle laughter; I imagine it would be very unnerving to have a client start chuckling during a treatment. Do they massage faces? Maybe I should get a face massage. Surely that's not a thing? I wonder what ... Oh, it's over. Half an hour gone by in about five seconds.

'Your right shoulder was incredibly knotty!' I always amaze masseuses with my knottiness.

'Was it?'

'Yeah, really knotty. I'll leave you to get ready, but no rush.'

Reader, I rushed. I walk home in the rain, dazzled by the headlights of all the traffic that's clogging up Goddy since the road closed. I stop at the One Stop and get some cash out of the standalone cash machine inside, and buy £9 worth of sweets. Over the shoulder of the cashier, rows and rows of vodka and gin. 'Anything else?' 'Erm ...' Play the tape forward. 'Nah, that's all right, just the sweets, please.' Lovely sweets.

'How was it?' asks Mum.

'Yeah, great. They told me to drink a lot of water and said I was incredibly knotty.'

'Oh, they say that to everyone.'

'Yeah, I've always wondered if they do that. By the way, I bought Dad some Rolos. Oh, and she also said ...'

'DON'T PUT YOUR HEAD ON THAT CUSHION! You're all greasy!'

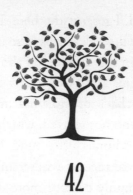

42

Peterborough hospital has become well swish since I was born there. It's also moved to a different part of the city, so technically I wasn't born 'there' any more, but still, it's pretty swanky. Car park is a bloody nightmare, though. Hinchingbrooke doesn't have a FibroScan machine, so I've been referred here.

'Okay, just lift your shirt up or take it off, whatever's comfortable,' says the nurse, 'and pop yourself on the table. Head up that end, feet down this end.'

'Thank you.'

'Did you get parked okay?'

'Eventually.'

'You just have to abandon your car somewhere in that car park.'

It's cold on the blue leathery examination table. I cross my hands over my stomach, that'll hide it, and look down at my red shoes. Very stylish. Hard to drive in, compared to trainers, quite heavy-footed; I kept revving in the car park and startling people, but I'll get used to them. I'm getting déjà vu from the flotation tank, as clear jelly is smeared on my torso, making me once again think of myself as a pork pie. Perhaps I was one in a past life. The FibroScan works its magic and I'm putting my shirt back on within a minute. My liver is back to normal size and not scarred, which is a relief. 'If it is bad news, the crematorium is just around the corner from the hospital,' Dad reassured me as I was setting off an hour ago.

'I feel lucky, I certainly deserve more damage, considering the last twenty years.' I don't mention that I think I've damaged my brain a bit, that when it's quiet I hear a buzzing sound, like wasps, or that I'm often startled by cars/people that don't exist in the corners of my vision.

'No, you don't deserve damage, no one deserves damage. How are you getting on with it all?'

'Well, I've gone from always drunk to almost always sober, but I don't really know how to live yet. I don't really know who ... I don't know ... I mean ... I was drunk for twenty years, I don't really know who I am. Yeah, I don't know.'

The nurse floats the idea that I could go back to Change Grow Live, a voluntary drug and alcohol misuse organisation with a centre in Huntingdon, which was called Inclusion last time I stopped going, and volunteer to talk to other people who are going through similar problems. She says it might help me as well. I think I'll look into that, in the new year; the new decade, which is only weeks away. Actually, I'd better concentrate on my own recovery before I jump ahead of myself. I'll try to sort the mess out in my head before I go near anyone else's. That can be my hobby.

I thank her and head home to help deck the halls. I know when I'm back in Godmanchester when the air becomes perfumed by wood burners. That, and the sign saying 'Godmanchester', and the fact that I'm familiar with the geography of the place.

'This tree has seen better days,' says Dad, having said the same last year, as we assemble, unfold, twist and turn, turn, turn the tower of green spikes until it's fully spruced. Mum won't abide a ratty tree. Dad's hurt his back hauling the garden waste wheelie bin around. 'It's really bad this time – this must be what it feels like to be old,' he says. We decide to have a cup of tea. Mum and Dad have had the windows cleaned for Christmas. Dad offered the window cleaner a drink and he asked for green tea, which caused quite some panic. Mum had to make it. She ended up putting Sweetex in it on autopilot. It reminded me of when I offered the Sky man a drink in London and he asked if I had any mango juice. I was fresh out.

'I'm going to have a mince pie.'

'Should you ought to, Paul?'

'I don't know, should I?'

'No.'

'Oh, I was sure I was about to have one.'

'I'm just looking after you,' Mum says, and jiggles his belly. I follow him to the kitchen and we sneak a bit of cheese.

After tea he rushes back to his study to finish up balancing the books for various family members. Soon that study will be home to the results of my next adventure. You see, I've ordered a load of clay from Amazon to make a bust of Dad's head. Michelangelo, carve your heart out, there's a new sculptor in town. I've always wanted to be crafty. We went to the Godmanchester Christmas Market the other day, which is full of crafty bits and bobs, as well as mulled wine, coffee, chilli sauce stand (maybe I'll become a chilli sauce guy one day), face-painting and cakes and the Mayor, looking like Santa in his big red smock. Mum bought another wooden stag. Mum has so many stags in the house. It's worrying. 'I've got hundreds, haven't I!' she beamed earlier, while looking around the living room. 'I bet I've got fifteen in this room alone.' I counted twenty-six. She said all this while wearing her stag jumper. 'You look nice, Mum,' I told her, pointing to her top. We both looked at Dad to see if he would say 'Mum looks nice', and he soon clocked that something was expected of him.

'What? Oh. Yes. Well, you always look nice.'

'That's a feeble excuse for not saying so!' Mum replied, before rushing off to deal with some mini sausages. So, yes, I thought about making a model of a stag, but 28 stags (26 + the one from the Christmas market + a home-made clay stag) in one room would perhaps be overkill. Much better to make Dad's head; we've only got one of those at the minute anyway.

It's tomorrow now. The clay's arrived (heavy!) but I realise I need some paint and some carving tools, so I walk into Huntingdon. There's a craft shop called Patches, where the Waitrose used to be before they closed it down. It's so warm today. Eleven degrees celsius. I try not to wear the big coat but I fail, it's just too hardwired: December = coat. I'm sweating by the time I trip on the step and fall through the door of the craft shop. There's one other shopper, an older lady in a grey parka looking at crochet hooks. Singalong sixties hits play through a little radio. It's oppressively cosy. I think if I stay any longer my blood will turn into wool. I've made a miscalculation coming here. It's a lovely shop, don't get me wrong, but it's quickly apparent it specialises in haberdashery.

In fact, that's what the sign outside says, but until just now, in the shop, I didn't know what haberdashery meant. Looks like I'll have to pretend to look at some buttons for a few minutes. 'Cheers, then!' I shout to nobody as I walk back out into the brutal, mild winter to perch on the stone bench opposite Boots, all bunched up like a big S, and search on my phone for a solution.

The following day I'm out for a walk when a lorry speeds through a deep puddle and drowns me on the pavement. 'Cheers, mate,' I shout, or something to that effect. I drip into my parents' house to find Dad's jeans on the kitchen floor in a wet heap – the same thing happened to him in the same spot about five minutes ago. I also see that Father Amazon has been and delivered the crafting tools and paint for the clay that's been warming by the navy blue AGA. Today one of my Very British Problems tweets is being beamed across Piccadilly Circus on the big flashy advertising board. I should really go and look at it in person, but I'd rather be making Clay Dad. And he won't make himself. It's the perfect opportunity: Real Dad is at the kitchen table with his big dictionary, drying off while tackling a Codeword. Mum and I bring out the large plastic chopping board and the clay and join him. Now there's no need to use the photo I took of Dad, which he looked at and said, 'Yeah, thought so, still the same grey old git.' He didn't sound jokey when he said this, more just sad. He's never liked photos being taken of him, and he's not keen on unnecessary smiling. Mum always says, 'He's happy on the inside, aren't you Paul? PAUL? I said you're happy on the inside, aren't you?' Anyway, there's no need for a photo now because we've got the real thing modelling live for us, and the Codeword will keep him still. Mum and I set about the grey clay, which is a bit like depressed Play-Doh, and with no prior sculpting experience, set about making a head.

Mum's in charge of the ears and the nose, the delicate bits, I'm in charge of ripping and moulding, as her hands aren't strong enough any more for that kind of heavy lifting. In essence, I'm basically just in charge of rolling the clay into a sphere. Quite relaxing. Much like spreading rice on seaweed. It's good to get your hands dirty. However, it's not all fun and games: the tools I ordered are absolute pants, all bendy and pathetic, so we use a butter knife for intricate carving, which goes through the clay like, well, butter.

'It doesn't matter if it's not perfect, Mum, it can be a bit rough. The worse it is the more character it'll have.'

'I don't think you need to worry about it being perfect, Robert. I wouldn't worry about that at all. His eyes are a bit high. And you've forgotten to give him a chin.'

'Hang on, god, I've just squashed the ears, pass the knife, please,' I say with the authority of a surgeon (you would not want me performing surgery on you – see the clay head for details).

'Look, Paul, what do you think? PAUL!'

Dad looks up like a shocked otter and points his head towards the work in progress. Then he tuts, raises his woolly eyebrows (very well replicated on the sculpture, I must say) and, seeking solace in the sturdy logic of puzzles, returns to his paper and sinks his eyebrows back into tray table position. Mum can't stop chuckling. 'You haven't given him any eyelids,' she notes. She's right, I have not. Oh well.

'It's good, this chopping board, isn't it?'

'Yeah, it's pretty good, Mum. Right, shall we leave him to dry?'

'Yes, hang on, I'll put him on a plate.'

'A Spode plate? No, you might ruin it. How about putting him on a Tupperware lid?'

'That's a good idea. We'll paint him tomorrow.' Mum switches to a whisper. 'It does actually look quite a lot like him! Bless him.'

We all retreat to the lounge for tea and shortbread shaped like mini Christmas trees. Mum reunites with her iPad.

'What are you thankful for this Christmas, Mum?' Mum lowers her iPad and thinks carefully.

'That we're all alive and healthy.'

'What about my back?' Dad chips in.

'Well, be thankful you've got a back,' Mum replies, while raising the iPad back to her face.

'What are you thankful for, Dad?'

'I'm still alive,' he says, with the intonation of a question, as if seeking confirmation.

'You could've said because you've still got me!' says Mum.

'Well, that's a given.' He takes a sip of tea from his reindeer mug. 'I got the moose head and the reindeer working, by the way.'

'Good. Come and look at this video,' Mum says, beckoning me to her bit of sofa. 'Come and look at this daft cat.' So I do, and Dad puts his glasses on and looks too, and the daft cat has us in stitches.

Later, while Mum and Dad watch *The Lion King* and I do some work on the laptop, Mark calls, sounding shaken up.

'What's up?'

'Well ... we ... erm ... we were just in Nando's, me, Jane and James, and this guy was causing trouble, throwing stuff around the restaurant and spitting at staff.'

'God. That's terrible.'

'Yeah, well, he storms out, then we hear this massive bang. He's come back with a sledgehammer and he's smashing up the window. As soon as we hear that first bang everyone just jumps up. I mean, the place is full of kids. He's banging it and then glass sprays over half the restaurant.'

'Oh my god, did the police come?'

'Yeah, the police came. We were all led out the back. We'd just done our Christmas shopping. We'd usually go to McDonald's after shopping, but fancied Nando's for a change.'

'So you're back home now?'

'Yeah, back home now.'

'Is James okay?'

'Yeah, he's okay. I asked if he wanted to go to McDonald's when we left Nando's but he just wanted to come straight home. He's on the floor now, doing some press-ups.'

I'm shocked, and relieved that everyone is okay. It reminds me how quickly things can go wrong, and how it's important to embrace and cherish the status quo while the quo-ing is good.

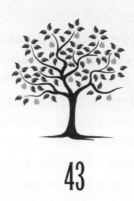

43

Hello. You're just in time to join the thrill ride that is vinegaring a ham. Have you ever vinegared a ham? I'll take your silence as a no.

'The ham's here!' Dad shouts, as the doorbell sounds. I imagine a ham standing at the door in a scarf with a suitcase and presents. Instead it's in a cardboard box being held by a human man. 'Ooh, that's a lovely box,' says Mum. 'Good for packing things up from your house!'

Any effort at veganism has gone out the window. Lunch is pretty much just party snacks now, eaten at the kitchen table with a knife and fork. I went to Big Tesco yesterday and filled a trolley with mini Kievs, ham and cheese croquettes, mini duck spring rolls with hoisin sauce – all sorts of battered and filo'd beige delights, and the quadrant of dips – three white and one pink. So tasty! Too tasty! I've started doing an online weight loss thing with Lauren (personal trainer Lauren, not masseuse Lauren), keeping a food, sleep, steps, hydration diary which she advises on. It's going to be embarrassing putting, 'Lunch: 8 chicken Kievs' on a spreadsheet. I questioned whether December was the right month to start this sort of thing, excuses excuses.

'There's never a good time to start,' Lauren says. 'Holidays, birthdays, there's always something that gets in the way. Now is as good a time as any. You can still enjoy Christmas, Rob! I certainly will. It's no problem. If you can start some small habits now, though, like logging your food and going for walks, it'll be so beneficial. You deserve to treat yourself well.' So I've started doing that. I must say, I hate logging my food. It's admin, and seems to take a little bit of joy from each meal, but the less I eat, the less I have to do it, so that's ideal, really. Also, I know how to lose weight: eat less, move more. But knowing that hasn't ever got me any slimmer; just like knowing not drinking means staying sober has never, on its own, kept me sober. So I've decided to stop knowing it all and follow Lauren's advice. Cottage cheese and popcorn will be my friends over Christmas. But also ham. I had to take some full body shots by the blankest bit of wall I can find and send them to Lauren. Front, sides and back, standing straight and gormless. I look like a podgy criminal (one of Michael Jackson's lesser-known hits) newly arrested for robbing a pie factory. A giant thumb in sports kit.

Dad fetches the industrial Sarson's from the shed. It's practically a petrol can of vinegar. Now, before I get in serious legal trouble, it's not technically the ham that gets vinegared, it's the calico ham bag. While the bag's soaking in water and vinegar, you wrap the ham in greaseproof paper, then stretch a net over it to keep the paper in place. Then you wring out the calico bag and put the ham inside it. This means it'll keep for longer, until well into January, by which time you'll never want to see ham again. It's a preservation thing, nothing to do with flavour. It'll also make the fridge burp vinegar at you every time you open the door, like opening a giant jar of pickled onions. Before we do this, though, we taste-test a couple of slices, hacked off using the big bendy ham knife which Dad keeps in a special long box in what I term the 'novelty cutlery' drawer – the drawer with the kebab skewers and the silver fish bottle opener that everyone had in the 1990s and the boiled-egg slicer. A ragtag bunch of mavericks. The A-Team of the kitchen implement world.

'Ooh, I just had a taste sensation!' says Mum. 'Here, chew one of these and then eat a bit of ham,' she continues, handing me a large chewable vitamin C tablet. I do as I'm told.

'What do you think?'

Truthfully? It's a unique recipe, for sure. It'd certainly hold scurvy at bay. But I'm not sure about it. It's a bit like . . . orangey ham.

'Mmm, yeah, lovely.'

'Isn't it!'

For our family, this is as much a Christmas tradition as decorating the tree. Once we've vinegared the ham bag, the festive season is officially under way. Stand by. There we go. It only takes about a minute, so it's done now. It's not the most exciting adventure, to be honest; I just really like saying 'ham bag'.

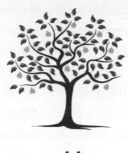

44

'Hello, my love, need any help with your packing?'

'Nah, I'll be fine thanks. Cheers, though.'

'Is this you all ready for Christmas, then?'

'Yeah, just about getting there! You?'

'Few bits and bobs left to do, but yeah . . . getting there.'

Pause.

'Busy day today.'

'I work from home, so not too bad. You?'

'It's been quite quiet today, probably get busy later. What is it you do?'

'I'm a writer, mostly, technology stuff. Gadgets and whatnot.'

'Oh I see . . . it's all robots now, isn't it? Everything's being done by robots.'

'Yeah, all sounds a bit scary, doesn't it?' She must have heard the bloke who walked past me at the end of the ghost tour in Cambridge, too; the one invested in building a killer robot army.

'Yeah, if we're not careful we'll end up like in *The Predator*.'
I think she means *Terminator*, but much of a muchness.

'That'd be a sod, wouldn't it?'

'Oh, it'd be awful. They wanna watch it. Yeah … I don't trust them at all. Club Card?'

'Yep, thank you.'

'Well, if I don't see you before, have a good Christmas, my love.'

'Thank you, you too, have a good one!'

'Cheers, then, seeya. Hello my love, any help with your packing?'

The supermarket is a strange place in December. Full of overwhelmed people walking around in a daze, leaving their trolleys at odd angles, all thinking about the next thing they have to remember to do instead of the task in hand. They stand catatonic in front of a wall of cheeses, thinking, 'Must remember to pick up some cinnamon.' Then off they go, to the spices, while trying to figure out what they need to make a 'third ox costume' suitable for a school nativity (I was meant to be a sheep in a nativity play. Mum dressed me up as a badger). Or they're just wishing December was over, wondering how they're going to pay for the whole thing. It's a nightmare getting home. Traffic in Godmanchester has been chock-a-block since the new A14 opened a few weeks ago.

I think I'm going to stop trying to be an adventurer now. I never was one. You probably noticed round about the 'Going For a Sandwich' adventure. The main block that I've stumbled over every time I've tried to navigate over or around the stumbling block is: I'm just not adventurous enough. This is confirmed by Spotify telling me my most listened-to bands of the decade are The Beatles and Oasis. Not adventurous for big adventures, anyway. I'd rather have ten thousand little things on my bucket list than fifty bonanza ones. Besides, a lot of clever people seem to agree in various pithy quotes that going looking for happiness is the surest way not to find it (I'm doing that reverse engineering thing again, aren't I?). The good thing about quotes is there's at least one to justify you in almost any behaviour or opinion.

This seismic news is all a bit out of the blue, I know, like when Forrest Gump decided to stop running, but I'm okay with being plain. You've got to accentuate the adequate. It is what it is. It feels like this year has been a long training exercise in how to best deal with the next breakdown. I've certainly put on a decent show for Instagram. I've firmly identified my comfort zone. Why do we think 'comfort zone' is a bad thing, anyway? If you were in a place with a door that said 'Comfort Zone' on it, you'd go straight in, wouldn't you? Why should you live each day as if it's your last? What an awful punishment. So hectic. Surely better to live each day as if there's a million more ahead?

Speaking of doors, Dad comes bustling in the front one, arms full of lever arch files, whooshing in the cold with him. It's so blustery out there, wind flashing across the grass in waves, the lawn a duvet cover being whipped shipshape. Light rain sputters in the air, like the fizz at the top of a glass of champagne. Dad's been to Peterborough to pick up some-one's accounts. He does a lot of work, for a retired person. He does more work than me. I help him wrap Mum's 'secret' present while she's having her nails done. She saw an advert for a Dyson hairdryer last night. 'Mum said she wondered if Santa would get her one, so I went to John Lewis this morning while I was in town,' says Dad. I fetch some gold wrapping paper from the wardrobe. Dad and I share an inability to wrap gifts in a way that doesn't leave them looking like they've been mauled by leopards. I've already attempted to wrap Dad's present, a Jo Malone aftershave, described as having a scent which involves 'midnight rain', a 'carnal touch of cumin and chilli leaves' and which is 'humid with moss'. He's going to smell like a sexy curry that's been left in the garden. We have a good run at wrapping the Dyson. It all goes wrong at one point when Dad turns like a startled collie to stare at a plane flying past the study window, letting go of the shiny paper as he does. We soldier on, then admire our work. 'Mum's a lot better at wrapping,' he says.

I'm on my third day of walking over ten thousand steps. Well, I've completed two days; today I'm up to about three thousand so far. I'm on my way to the polling station at Judith's Field, next to the College of Animal Welfare. Polling was in the actual college at the last vote, at the start of the summer, while the pavilion at Judith's Field was being renovated. I can't remember what we were voting for back then, but thanks to Instagram I can see that I took a photograph of a life-size model of a horse, complete with the caption: 'This guy was at the polling station #horse'. Six likes. I can see that Mum commented, 'Would love him in the garden'. I also recall it was hot. I saw a woman jogging in full kit while eating a Calippo. What a hero. Take away the jogging, and you've got the perfect day right there.

No ice lollies in sight today, it's raining cats and dogs. A chill wind blows, too, wrapping around my cheeks like old, cold hands. I keep checking my pocket for my polling card, like you do a passport at the airport, even though it says quite clearly on the polling card that I don't need it. I know ten thousand steps is an arbitrary number, but it's better than my daily average of about eleven. I've slept really well the past two nights. 'It's amazing what a bit of fresh air can do,' Lauren assured me. I'm already thinking, 'If ten thousand steps makes me feel fresh, imagine what twenty thousand would do!'

Mum, Dad and I are having our work Christmas party today, lunch at The Black Bull, which has recently turned itself into a steakhouse-cum-ribshack. 'Inviting your account-ant to your office party?' Dad asks, surprised. 'Someone's got to pay!' I reply. Nah, it's my treat, least I can do. Whether it be made up of relations, friends or animals, thank god for family. There's a queue of dripping Godmanchester residents at the polling station, shaking brollies and whipping off hoods. We all confirm to one another through eye-rolls and puffed-out cheeks and exhales that it's certainly a rainy day. I approach the desk of four volunteers, as usual, with trepidation. How many of the four should I attempt to make eye contact with? I manage two and a half.

'Erm . . . Temple? Robert Temple?'

'Okay . . . what's your address, Thomas?'

I say my address.

'Here it is. Temple . . . Robert?'

'Yes, that's right '

'Okay, here you go, just over there please.'

I take my ballot paper to the little raised table, grab the pencil on the string and study the five options for much longer than necessary. Putting a cross in the box, panicking that I'm meant to do a tick instead of a cross, then seeing that no, I was right to do the cross, I then study the thing for another minute or two to check I haven't accidentally written 'WILLY' or 'ELEPHANT' across it. All seems in order.

'I just pop it in here, do I?'

'Yes.'

I carefully slot my folded ballot paper into the black cube, certain that I've just posted my wallet into a postbox. Then I walk out feeling like a hero. I may have just saved this beautiful damn country. Someone had to do it. I even give a little nod to passers-by on their way to cast their votes, which are now meaningless because I have settled the matter. The ground is slick with layers of mushed-up leaves and mud, with the occasional patch of pavement, slippery as ice. It's as precarious as how I imagine walking on a giant lasagne would be, the top layer desperate to slide off at any moment. I treat myself to a ride on the mini zip wire in the park. The wind chucks a big wet leaf in my face.

'You're definitely looking thinner since you've been walking,' Mum says. I've actually gained two pounds in the last two days, but it's nice of her to say. I take any form of light exercise as an excuse to double my calorie intake, which at the minute is mostly delivered in the form of crackers, from a variety tin I bought from Tesco that says 'Have yourself a merry little Christmas' on the lid (surely 'Have a cracking Christmas' or 'Christmas crackers' would have been better?). I'm using these crackers, every time I enter the kitchen, to dip into anything wet and scoopable from the fridge. Crackers: edible plates. Like most people in December, I'm also eating a lot of individually wrapped chocolates, as well as the contents of an Advent calendar (I'm close to forty). I wish you got more than one chocolate a day in an Advent calendar. Even though I've plenty of chocolates in the cupboard, it just tastes so much better when they have to be pulled through a tiny cardboard door.

Walking. It almost always lifts my mood. A long march with favourite tunes seems to kill off self-pity and self-indulgent negativity; plodding around Godmanchester reminds me that life is pretty good. It's a wonderful place. My spirits aren't even dampened when my feet savagely are, when I try to run across a flooded Portholme Meadow (it's so large), leaving me shin-deep in freezing water, squishy grass and mud. This must be what it's like to stand in a blocked toilet, I think, horrifically. But yeah, those scientists weren't wrong about endorphins, were they? That's good stuff. I should let them know. They're right about medicine, too. Anxiety is real. It's a natural reality; a useful emotion that can get out of whack and start inhibiting you. Confidence is the trick, the illusion, and if you can get a bit nearer to it with pills, I'm happy to swallow them. Mix endorphins with meds and there's a cocktail that does the same trick as a couple of martinis. For me, anyway. Still, I've been here before, thrilled about a new magic cure (I tend to discover the walking/running version of the cure at the ends and starts of years), then sucker-punched into bed for a week.

The family-run Black Bull, opposite the war memorial, has lots of new high-backed red leather chairs, a blackboard with a chalk drawing of a cow divided up into all its edible bits, and menus on rough beige paper written in cowboy/wanted poster font (Slab Serif? Oswald? Bree Serif? I think it might be one of the serifs) attached to clipboards. Yee-har. Oh look, they do an eating challenge. A 40 oz 'Quadzilla' Burger; finish it in forty-five minutes and the price goes from £50 to £20. Fifty quid? Doesn't seem worth the risk. We chose The Black Bull, as the Godmanchester Living Facebook page has been full of praise for the new set-up. We sit at a table in front of the fireplace. A radio station plays songs and shouts adverts through the wall-mounted speakers, tucked away amongst fairy lights. Mum and Dad have scampi in a basket, in this case a little metal shopping basket; I have rib-eye steak, not in a basket but on a chopping board, although my chips are in a basket, with a little pan of Stilton sauce on the side. So many non-plate-based accessories. They must have a funny-shaped dishwasher. I want to order a side salad, just to see if it comes in a mini wheelbarrow, or perhaps some extra onion rings stuffed in the boot of a tiny car.

'Weird song to eat lunch to on a Friday afternoon, isn't it?' says Natasha, the new landlady, as the 'Macarena' soundtracks her walk to the kitchen. I like it here. We have a cracking time. Mum tickles Dad to get him to smile for my photo-graph. I pay the bill – I still get a small thrill from paying for my parents' meal; it feels like when I was small and Dad would sit me on his knee in the car and let me steer the car on the driveway – and we enter a raffle for an Alzheimer's char-ity, then we coat up and walk home through the graveyard.

'I don't know,' I say, 'big shop, long walk, vote, zip wire, steak lunch . . . what a day!'

'Yes, you're really living the dream, aren't you?' Mum replies, with joyous sincerity. I probably am living the dream. Maybe life is about learning to be content with what you can be bothered to achieve. And being thankful for peaceful days.

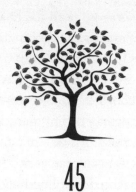

45

Christmas Day comes and goes in a blizzard of cranberry sauce and party poppers, and cracker jokes and Dad – reluctantly wearing his pink paper hat while permanently washing up at the sink; red Shloer, Lisa's lovely boozeless trifle, piles of various-sized spoons plonked on tables and work surfaces, Pete's red Christmas trousers and new socks in boxes of three, made by Pringle and Ted Baker and Jeep ('Jeep do socks?!') lying about the place. 'Are these your socks or mine?' Dad's on big bin bag duty for the wrapping that everyone thinks just magically disappears somewhere along the journey from gift to floor. Everyone ratchets their jolly moods up a notch. People sneak around the house holding scissors and Sellotape, speed-wrapping presents cross-legged on spare room carpets. Mum urged us to remind her not to forget to take the turkey out of the shed, which nobody did, but she remembered anyway. We wear festive clothes and at first do a lot of standing instead of sitting, later followed by a lot of sitting. My phone plays Christmas carols out of its speakers (which are so clear there's no need for Dad to find his mini Bluetooth speaker this year), but choirs are a bit hectic (and some are downright sinister) for eating, so we put on Bublé.

I treat myself to a spray of the aftershave Lisa bought me for my birthday last month; it's almost too nice to use, but it's Christmas! The Christmas pudding flames nicely. For years it never did, as Mark and I had watered down the brandy so much. We all take turns to play James at Mario Kart. The yo-yo proves a big hit; invented four hundred years before Jesus (maybe Jesus had a yo-yo? Note to self: look into this), and still entertaining whole families on the cusp of 2020. Who needs a Nintendo Switch when you've got a plastic disc on a string? Goop emails me a newsletter with the subject line 'It's Goop to Have You', which makes me want to stop using my body brush.

Then that stagnant time between Boxing Day and New Year's Eve swamps us, that time when every day feels a bit 'Sunday cocktail-shakered with a tot of Monday'. I think they call it Twixmas, now. Everyone's full. I suspect my blood type is currently 'cheese'. Time feels like headphones that've knotted in your pocket. I bet even Scrooge fought to keep his jolly new personality going once he was sick of parsnips and stollen. Then again, he probably didn't have a new rose-gold Fitbit Charge 3 that he bought on the cheap on Boxing Day waiting for him to pick up at the St Ives Waitrose. I spend the days making sandwiches filled with so many different things they end up tasting of nothing. Before we know it, Jools Holland is telling us it's ten seconds till January. Almost time to throw away the leftover sprouts we've had cling-filmed in a little bowl in the fridge since Christmas Day.

The leaves have deserted the trees and all the apples are

gone. Well, not gone. They're in the shed, or mashed up and in the freezer. And we've got a few non-cooking apples in the fruit bowl, which I enjoy eating with a knife – makes me feel like Crocodile Dundee. Mum and Dad and I start the new decade with a walk into town. It's a very mild day in the Fens, but we're dressed for mountains. It's nice to be outside. We stop off at Caffè Nero. Big-band music blasts from all corners. Dad talks about his New Year's resolution. 'I'm not going to eat sugar any more,' he declares, between bites of *stroopwafel*.

'Remember when we went to Spain, Janet? I was 13 stone 8!'

'You were still overweight then!'

'That's not much encouragement.'

'I've been married to you for forty-five years, and I've heard this day in, day out.'

'It's a good job I don't get hurt feelings.'

'It's my way of looking after you,' she says, passing Dad the Sweetex she keeps in her handbag. 'You're still alive, aren't you?'

Dad starts to tell me a story about a bad hotel experience they had one New Year's Eve, but Mum cuts him off saying he's told the story a million times. Mum carries on telling the story to its conclusion. I want to keep working hard at staying well for them, and for myself. They've stuck me back together. I'd like to try harder at being cheery. It takes less energy than being a curmudgeon. I need to stop worrying so much about trying to live in the now. It must be impossible, otherwise Scrooge would've needed just one ghost rather than three. Living in the now is just a convenient way to ignore your mistakes. How do you learn anything if you live without regret? Especially if the regrets are your own fault ... If you simply forget about them and your past, surely you run a strong risk of remaining a tosser? It's probably time I moved out of my parents' home and attempted to be an adult again. I'll wait until spring, when the crumble runs out.

'This is my second completely sober December, you know?'

'You're not going to make up for that in January, are you?' asks Mum, wearily.

'I hope not. I think I might get back into jogging. If only to get the steps done quicker. Get myself nice and trim for the summer.'

'Sounds like a good idea,' says Dad as he cleans up the table, tidying crumbs and neatly stacking cups and saucers so they're easy for the staff to take away.

'What's your New Year's resolution, Mum?'

'Oh, I don't bother with any of that. New Year's resolutions are just last year's failures. Right, shall we go home? We could watch *Bridget Jones* again.'

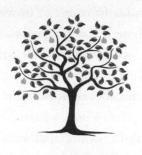

AFTERWORD

The *There Or Thereabouts English Dictionary* (written by me and kept in my head, you can't find it in print) defines an Afterword as 'a bit of a conclusion often found at the back of a book' – the final ingredient that brings the meat of the tale together, quickly reheating everything on the plate, much like a gravy. So you can relax: you've come to the right place (if you were looking for an Afterword/gravy analogy).

Right! [*slaps knees*] What have I learned? I'll deploy another food analogy, if I may. After all, there's nothing like whipping up a quick one of those to clumsily disguise what in hindsight I fear will appear to be quite an obvious message (like on *Masterchef*, when they try to disguise the fact that they've just made a bog-standard cheese on toast by decorating it with some micro herbs). Here we go.

Life is like a sausage sandwich: you do pretty much know what you're going to get. Yes, the unexpected does happen, but come on, all your days, on the whole, are quite similar, aren't they? That's just how life with all its routines and little boring necessities works for most of us regular schlubs. You make your sandwich each day pretty much how you made it yesterday. Now, in a sausage sandwich (life), you can have red sauce (doing lots of things) or brown sauce (doing nothing). I've discovered that for the most pleasant sausage sandwich (life), I like to have a mix of both sauces (you get the picture). Stick that in your pipe (mind) and smoke it (consider it). Over the past year, I've also recognised that when my sausage sandwich (life) gets too much for me to digest, I have a tendency to wrap part of it up in tinfoil (tiresome dad jokes) and put it away in the back of the fridge (deeply repress it). Then life goes to shit. Sorry, I mean, then the sausage sandwich goes mouldy.

The trouble I'm having is, how much is all this really a revelation to me? I have an ominous feeling that I've discovered all of this before, in one way or another, at the end of most adult years I've had. As Peter Cook said, 'I have learned from my mistakes, and I am sure I can repeat them exactly'. Mind you, I must have experienced a tiny bit of evolution these past twelve months: I spent a lot less of it in bed than previous years. Typically, I'm so indecisive I can't decide what I've learned.

By the time I'm ninety-two, after I've ruined plenty of breakfasts, I'll have the perfect sausage sandwich recipe all worked out, and I'll discover I knew exactly how I liked it all along, and that I should've enjoyed it while I could still chew. I *think* I know what I'm talking about, maybe? Ah well, doesn't matter. Anyway, hungry now. Cheerio.

ACKNOWLEDGEMENTS

My love and thanks to Juliet Mushens and Hannah Boursnell (best of luck for your next adventure, Hannah) and everyone at Mushens Entertainment and Little, Brown. All those partial to Very British Problems (@SoVeryBritish). The good people of Hinchingbrooke Hospital for repeatedly fixing me. Mother Nature for cooking up such a variety of tasty apples. And to Mum and Dad, family and friends, and everyone who joined me on a frightfully mild adventure.

Additional credits: *Tragically I was an Only Twin: The Complete Peter Cook* by Peter Cook (Century, 2002); *Willy Wonka & the Chocolate Factory* by Roald Dahl, directed by Mel Stuart (Wolper Pictures Ltd, 1971); *The Gun Seller* by Hugh Laurie (Soho Press, 1997); 'Teddy Bear' from *When We Were Very Young* by A. A. Milne (Methuen & Co Ltd, 1924); *The Secret Diary of Adrian Mole, Aged 13¾* by Sue Townsend (Penguin, 2002).